BBQ Recipe Book

70 Of The Best Ever Healthy Barbecue Recipes...Revealed!

Samantha Michaels

Table of Contents

Publishers Notes

Disclaimer

This publication is intended to provide helpful and informative material. It is not intended to diagnose, treat, cure, or prevent any health problem or condition, nor is intended to replace the advice of a physician. No action should be taken solely on the contents of this book. Always consult your physician or qualified health-care professional on any matters regarding your health and before adopting any suggestions in this book or drawing inferences from it.

The author and publisher specifically disclaim all responsibility for any liability, loss or risk, personal or otherwise, which is incurred as a consequence, directly or indirectly, from the use or application of any contents of this book.

Any and all product names referenced within this book are the trademarks of their respective owners. None of these owners have sponsored, authorized, endorsed, or approved this book.

Always read all information provided by the manufacturers' product labels before using their products. The author and publisher are not responsible for claims made by manufacturers.

Manufactured in the United States of America

Introduction

Just because you are trying to lose weight doesn't mean you actually need to forsake your favorite foods. Plus it also doesn't mean that when summer is here you only need to eat salads or steamed fish.

Did you know when trying to lose weight eating meals cooked on a barbecue can help you to achieve your goals?

Most people of course when the words "barbecue" are said will immediately think of warm summer evenings enjoying great food and drink with their friends and family. However by choosing to barbecue their food they are actually making a subconscious decision to eat more healthily.

Through barbecuing you will find yourself actually eating less fat. This is because when you choose to cook meat or fish on a barbecue you only need to provide a light coating of oil to the food to prevent it from sticking to the grill. Whereas when frying the same food you will use considerably more oil.

Another reason why barbecuing food is much better for you when losing weight is that it has a much lower calorie count. So of course the fewer calories being consumed means that you won't have to burn off so many when exercising. Yet you will still find that you can still eat the same amount of food.

As well as helping to reduce the amount of calories and fat you consume by grilling food on a barbecue you are actually reducing the chances of you developing such diseases as diabetes, high blood pressure, heart disease or a stroke.

Another benefit of actually grilling food on a barbecue is that it helps the food retain many of the nutrients, vitamins and minerals that our bodies need to function properly. So of course in turn this helps it to also eliminate such things as free radicals from it that can cause us to retain fat rather than lose it.

Certainly when it comes to cooking vegetables you will find putting them on the barbecue more beneficial to you than boiling or steaming them. This is because grilling does actually help them to retain as many vital nutrients that would normally be drained out of them.

Finally of course those who choose to grill food on a barbecue find that the food does actually taste better. This is because more of the foods natural flavor is retained.

Of course when it comes to cooking on a barbecue there are some recipes that may look and taste great, but may not help you in achieving your weight loss goals or help you to lead a much healthier lifestyle. However in this book with provide details of 70 healthy barbecue recipes you may want to consider trying.

Chapter 1 – Healthy Meat Recipes for the Barbecue

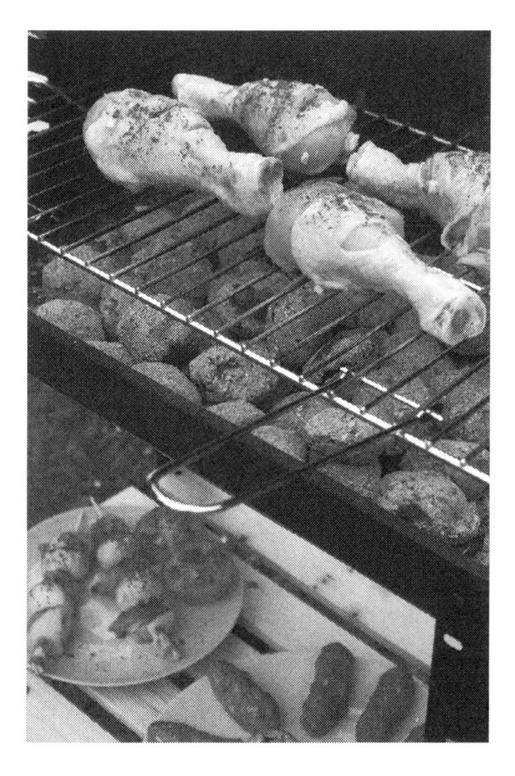

Recipe 1 – Unbelievable Chicken

This particular recipe doesn't require long to prepare and still produces very healthy but delicious tasting food. Each serving of this recipe provides a person with 337 calories and only 16.4g of fat.

Ingredients

6 Skinless Boneless Chicken Breasts
6 Tablespoons Olive Oil
60ml Cider Vinegar
3 Tablespoons Coarse Ground Mustard
3 Garlic Cloves Minced
Juice Of 1 Lime

Juice of ½ Lemon
110grams Brown Sugar
1 ½ Teaspoons Salt
Freshly Ground Black Pepper To Taste

Instructions

1. In a large bowl combine together the cider vinegar, mustard, garlic, lime and lemon juice, brown sugar, salt and pepper. Then whisk into this the olive oil and add chicken turning it over several times to ensure all sides of the breasts is covered in the marinade. Now cover the bowl over and place in the refrigerator for at least 8 hours. However it is best if you choose to leave it to marinate in the sauce overnight.

2. Just before you take the chicken out of the refrigerator you should heat up the barbecue. You will need to cook the chicken breasts on a medium to high heat so place the grill which has been lightly oiled about 4 to 6 inches above the heat source.

3. Once the barbecue has heated up you can now place the chickens on to the lightly oiled grill and cook for 6 to 8 minutes on each side, or when you insert a skewer into the thickest part of the chicken breast the juices that run out are clear. Any marinade that is left over should be discarded.

As soon as the chicken breasts are cooked serve with a fresh green salad.

Recipe 2 – Pineapple Chicken Tenders

This is a recipe that not only many children but adults will enjoy. The total number of calories that each serving offers you is just 160 and comes with only 2.2g of fat.

Ingredients

900grams Chicken Breasts (Cut Into Tenderloins Or Strips)
240ml Pineapple Juice
110grams Brown Sugar
80ml Light Soy Sauce

Instructions

1. In a small saucepan, which has been placed on a medium, put the pineapple juice, brown sugar and light soy sauce. Heat these ingredients through until they just begin to boil and then remove from the heat.

2. In a medium sized bowl place the chicken and then cover with the sauce you have just made. Cover the bowl and then place in the refrigerator to allow the chicken to marinate in the sauce for at least 30 minutes. The longer you leave the meat to marinate in the sauce then the more of the flavor will be absorbed by it.

3. Just before you take the chicken out of the refrigerator get the barbecue going and place the grill around 6 inches above the heat source. You will want to cook the chicken on a medium heat.

4. Whilst the barbecue is heating up thread the chicken on to some skewers. If you are using wooden ones make sure that you have soaked them in water for at least 30 minutes before using to prevent them from burning when placed on the barbecue.

5. After threading the chicken on to the skewers now lightly oil the grill just before placing them on to the barbecue. You should be cooking each piece of chicken on each side for at least 5 minutes.

If you are not sure if the chicken is ready pierce the thickest part of the meat with another skewer and if the juices inside run clear the chicken is cooked and ready to serve. Be careful and watch the chicken a lot as it cooks very quickly.

Recipe 3 – Greek Lamb Kebabs

As well as the meat being very lean, lamb also takes on some amazing flavors when cooked on a barbecue.

Ingredients

400grams Lean Lamb (Cut Into Cubes)
1 Lemon Cut Into Wedges
12 Bay Leaves

1 Large Courgette Sliced
1 Red Pepper Cut Into Chunks

Marinade

Olive Oil
Sprinkling Of Dried Oregano
Squeeze Of Lemon Juice

Instructions

1. If you are using wooden skewers place these in a flat dish with some water and leave for at least an hour.

2. Whilst the skewers are soaking in the water you can start cutting up the lamb, courgette and pepper ready for then threading on to the skewers.

3. About 15 minutes before you remove the skewers from the water you should get the barbecue heated up. Make sure that you place the grill of the barbecue about 6 inches above the heat source, as you want to cook these lamb kebabs on a medium heat.

4. After threading the lamb, courgette and pepper on to the skewers alternately you need to brush them with the olive oil, oregano and lemon juice. So in a small bowl whisk together these ingredients and then brush the mixture over the kebabs.

5. Now place the kebabs on to the barbecue grill that you have lightly oiled and cook on each side for about 2 minutes each or until the lamb is cooked. The lamb shouldn't be cooked all the way through but should still look at little pink inside when cut.

6. Let the kebabs rest for a few minutes then serve with a crisp green salad, some couscous, potato wedges or some pitta bread.

Recipe 4 – Maple Garlic Marinated Pork Tenderloin

You may think that using maple syrup is going to be bad for you when trying to lose weight yet each serving of this dish contains just 288 calories and 4.9g of fat.

Ingredients

680grams Pork Tenderloin
2 Tablespoons Dijon Mustard
1 Teaspoon Sesame Oil
3 Garlic Cloves Minced
340grams (240ml) Maple Syrup
Freshly Ground Black Pepper To Taste

Instructions

1. Into a large bowl combine together the mustard, garlic, sesame oil and maple syrup and whisk thoroughly.

2. Now in a shallow dish place the pork tenderloin and coat all sides evenly with the sauce you have just made. Then cover and place in the refrigerator to allow the pork to marinate in the sauce for at least 8 hours.

However if you want prepare it the day before and allow the meat to marinate in the sauce overnight. The longer you leave the pork in the marinade the more of it will be absorbed and the more tender and tasty the meat will be when cooked.

3. After removing the pork from the refrigerator get the barbecue heated up. It is best if you allow the pork to come up to room temperature before you then place it on the barbecue to cook. Also make sure that you put the grill of the barbecue at least 6 inches above the heat source, as you want to cook the meat on a low to medium heat. If you cook it on too high a heat the marinade will then burn.

4. Once the barbecue has heated up lightly oil the grill and then place the pork tenderloin on it. Any marinade you have left over should be poured into a saucepan and heated through for about minutes of a low to medium heat. This you will then use for basting the pork whilst it is cooking.

5. Cook the pork for around 15 to 25 minutes on the barbecue, making sure that you turn it over regularly. Only remove it from the barbecue once the inside of the meat is no longer pink. If you

would prefer not to cut the meat open whilst cooking then use a meat thermometer. The meat will be ready to eat when the interior temperature has reached 170 degrees Fahrenheit.

As soon as the pork is cook put to one side for a few minutes to rest before then carving and serving to your guests.

Recipe 5 – Marinated Turkey Breast

Turkey is one of the healthiest types of meat you can eat these days, as it is extremely lean. Each serving of this dish contains 317 calories and 6g of fat.

Ingredients

1400grams Boneless Turkey Breasts
2 Garlic Cloves Minced
1 Tablespoon Finely Chopped Fresh Basil
½ Teaspoon Freshly Ground Black Pepper
6 Whole Cloves
60ml Vegetable Oil
60ml Soy Sauce (Light Would Be Best)
2 Tablespoons Fresh Lemon Juice
1 Tablespoon Brown Sugar

Instructions

1. In a bowl combine together the minced garlic, basil and pepper, then rub all over the turkey breasts. Now into each end of the turkey breasts and in the middle insert a whole clove. Then place to one side in a shallow dish.

2. Next in to another bowl put the oil, soy sauce, lemon juice and brown sugar and whisk well to ensure that all these ingredients are mixed thoroughly. Once all these ingredients are well combined you should now pour them over the turkey breasts making sure that you turn the breasts over to ensure all sides of them are coated in the sauce. Then cover the dish over and place in the refrigerator for around 4 hours.

3. After you remove the turkey breasts from the refrigerator where they have been marinating in the sauce you should now get the barbecue heated up. It is important that you place the lightly oiled grill around 4 inches above the heat source, as you want to cook the turkey breasts on a high heat.

4. Once the barbecue has heated up you place the turkey breasts on to the lightly oiled grill and then close the lid. After about 15 minutes open the lid and turn the turkey breasts over and cook them for a further 15 minutes with the lid closed or until the juices run clear on the internal temperature of the breasts when a meat thermometer is inserted has reached 170 degrees Fahrenheit.

As for any leftover marinade this should be discarded.

Recipe 6 – Mojito Rubbed Chicken with Grilled Pineapple

This recipe certainly has a summer feel to it and yet is also extremely health. Each serving contains just 320 calories and 6g of fat.

Ingredients

4 Medium Sized Skinless And Boneless Chicken Breasts
2 Limes
1 Tablespoon Olive Oil
1 Medium Sized Pineapple (Weighing About 1600grams) Peeled and Cut Into ½ inch slices
32grams Loosely Packed Fresh Mint Leaves Chopped
Salt And Freshly Ground Black Pepper To Taste

Instructions

1. Heat up the barbecue placing the grill about 6 inches above the heat source, as you want to cook the food on a medium heat.

2. Whilst the barbecue is heating up take a meat mallet and pound the chicken which you may want to place between some sheets of plastic wrap or baking paper to they are ½ inch thick all over. Then place to one side ready for cooking.

3. Next take one of the limes and in to a bowl grate one teaspoon of zest and add to this 2 tablespoons of freshly squeezed juice from it. Then to this add the tablespoon of oil and mixed thoroughly.

4. Now take the slices of pineapple and brush them lightly with the mixture above and any sauce left over should be set to one side as you will need it for later. Now place the pineapple slices on to the grill of the barbecue that has been lightly oiled and cook on both sides for about 5 minutes each or until they are brown. Then when cooked remove from the heat and set to one side to serve with the chicken when cooked.

5. To the remaining sauce you now add the chopped mint leaves and then pat this marinade on to both sides of the chicken and then sprinkle them with some salt and pepper. Now place the chicken on the barbecue with the grill which has been lightly oiled placed 4 inches above the heat source as you will be cooking them on a high heat and cook for around 5 minutes turning them over once.

You should make sure that not only is the outside of the chicken brown but also the inside is no longer pink. The quickest way to see if the chicken is cooked through is to insert a skewer and see if the juices run clear.

6. After the chicken has been cooked place each one on to a place and serve with a slice of pineapple. As for the other lime this should be cut into wedges to serve with the pineapple and chicken.

Recipe 7 – Spiced Pork Tenderloin with Mango Salsa

As well as being very healthy each serving only containing 215 calories and 6g of fat this recipe is also very tasty and comes with a little kick.

Ingredients

2 x 450grams Pork Tenderloin
3 Tablespoons All Purpose Flour
1 Teaspoon Salt
1 Teaspoon Ground Cumin

1 Teaspoon Ground Coriander
½ Teaspoon Ground Cinnamon
½ Teaspoon Ground Ginger

Mango Salsa

2 Medium Sized Ripe Mangos Peeled And Coarsely Chopped
2 Medium Sized Kiwi Fruit Peeled And Coarsely Chopped
2 Tablespoons Seasons Rice Vinegar
1 Tablespoon Freshly Grated Peeled Ginger
1 Tablespoon Fresh Cilantro Leaves Minced

Instructions

1. Begin by preparing the Mango Salsa. To do this place the chopped mango, kiwi fruit into a medium sized bowl and then add to this the vinegar, ginger and cilantro leaves and mix well together with a spoon. As you won't be serving this straight away cover and place in the refrigerator.

2. Next you need to get the barbecue heated up and put the grill about 6 inches above the heat source as you will be cooking the pork on a medium heat. Whilst the barbecue is heating up you can now start to prepare the pork tenderloin.

3. Take the pork and cut each piece in half lengthwise. However you must cut the meat all the way through as you want to open each piece out and spread it flat. Then place each piece of pork between 2 sheets of plastic wrap and pound with a meat mallet or rolling pin until they are about ¼ inch thick then cut each piece into 4 other pieces.

4. Now take some waxed paper and on to this place the flour, cumin, coriander, ground ginger and salt and mix them together. Then place the pieces of flattened pork on to this mixture turning them over to ensure that all sides of the meat are evenly coated. Once you have done this you can now place the pork on to the grill and cook on each side for between 2 ½ and 3 minutes or until they are a light brown in color.

5. Once the pork is cooked meaning that it is now longer pink in color remove from barbecue place on to clean plates and serve with the Mango Salsa which you spoon over the top.

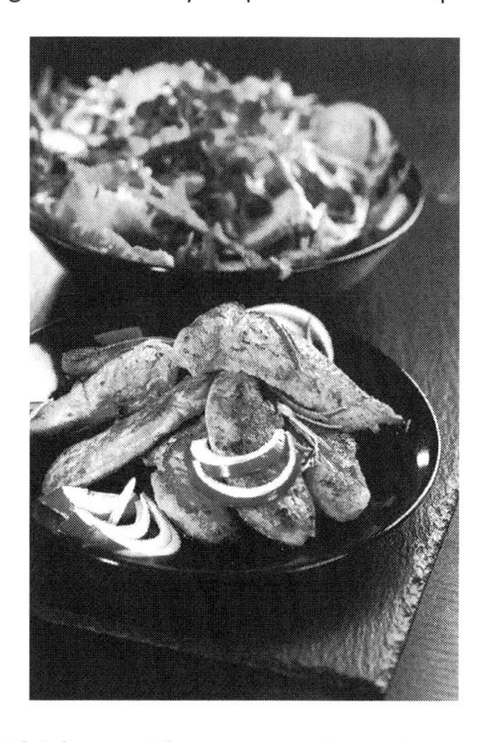

Recipe 8 – Chicken with Summer Squash

This is not only a very healthy option each serving containing only 225 calories but also low in fat on 8g per serving. If you prefer swap the squash for Eggplant.

Ingredients

4 Medium Sized Skinless And Boneless Chicken Thighs
4 Medium Sized Yellow Summer Squash Cut Lengthwise Into 4 Wedges
1 Lemon
1 Tablespoon Olive Oil
½ Teaspoon Salt
¼ Teaspoon Fresh Coarsely Ground Black Pepper
Handful Freshly Snipped Chives
Lemon Slices Grilled For Garnish

Instructions

1. In to a bowl combine 1 tablespoon of freshly grated lemon zest along with 3 tablespoons freshly squeezed lemon juice with oil, salt and pepper. Once fully combined put 2 tablespoons of this mixture into a bowl and set to one side.

2. To the sauce left in the bowl you now add the chicken thighs and cover then let them to marinate in this mixture for 15 minutes at room temperature. However if you would prefer the chicken thighs to absorb more of this wonderful marinade place them in the refrigerator for 30 minutes.

3. Whilst the chicken thighs are marinating you should now be heating up the barbecue. Place the grill of the barbecue 6 inches above the heat source, as you will want to cook the chicken thighs on a medium heat.

4. When the barbecue is ready take the chicken thighs out of the marinade and place them on to the lightly oiled grill. Any leftover marinade can now be thrown away. At the same time you place the chicken thighs on the barbecue also place the Summer Squash wedges and close the lid.

5. Cook the chicken and squash for about 10 to 15 minutes making sure that you turn them over regularly to prevent them burning. To test if the chicken is ready you insert a skewer in to the thickest part of the thigh. The chicken will be ready to eat when you see the juices from inside it running clear. As for the squash this should feel tender to the touch and be a golden brown color.

6. As soon as the chicken and squash are cooked place on clean plates and drizzle with the sauce you placed to one side earlier. Then sprinkle over the chives and place slice of grilled lemon on top.

Recipe 9 – Turkey Cutlets with Melon Salsa

The melon salsa served with the turkey cutlets helps to bring out other flavors within the meat. This is an extremely good recipe to try when attempting to lose weight as each serving only contains 185 calories.

Ingredients

Turkey Cutlets
4 Turkey Breast Cutlets
125grams Prosciutto Thinly Sliced
Salt And Freshly Ground Black Pepper

Melon Salsa

2 Limes
225gram Cantaloupe Chopped
225gram Honeydew Melon Chopped
75gram Pickling Cucumber Shredded
1 Jalapeno Chilli Deseeded And Finely Chopped
55gram Fresh Basil Leaves Chopped

Instructions

1. Get the barbecue heated up and place the grill on it about 6 inches above the heat source as you will be cooking the turkey cutlets on a medium heat.

2. Whilst the barbecue is heating up into a bowl mix 1 teaspoon of peel from one of the limes with 2 tablespoons of its juice. As for the other lime cut this into 4 wedges and put to one side for use when serving the cooked cutlets later.

3. Now add into the bowl with the lime juice and peel the melon, cucumber, and chilli and ¼ teaspoon of salt. Stir well to ensure that everything is well coated in the lime juice and then set to one side ready for placing on plates with the turkey later.

4. Just before you place the turkey cutlets on to the barbecue grill which has been lightly oiled sprinkle over each one some more lime peel along with some freshly grated black pepper. Then wrap around each one slices of the prosciutto and press it firmly against the turkey.

5. Now place the turkey on to the barbecue and cook for around 5 to 7 minutes or until the turkey meat is no longer pink in color. It is important that halfway through cooking your turn each turkey cutlet over ensure that the meat is cooked through evenly and also helps to prevent the prosciutto from becoming burnt.

6. Once the turkey cutlets are cooked transfer them to clean plates and serve them to your guests with some of the melon salsa and lime wedges.

Recipe 10 – Steak Sandwich with Grilled Onions

This is not only a very simple dish to prepare but also an extremely tasty one. Each sandwich contains just 210 calories and 3g of fat.

Ingredients

600grams Beef Flank Steak
1 Medium Sized Red Onion Cut Into 4 Thick Slices
60ml Soy Sauce
60ml Balsamic Vinegar
1 Tablespoon Brown Sugar
1 Teaspoon Fresh Thyme Leaves
¼ Teaspoon Freshly Ground Black Pepper
8 Slices Sourdough Bread
2 Medium Sized Ripe Tomatoes Sliced
1 Bunch Arugula With The Stems Removed

Instructions

1. Into a large resealable plastic bag pour the soy sauce, balsamic vinegar, thyme and pepper. Close and shake vigorously to ensure that all ingredients are combined well together.

2. Now into the bag put the steak and close the bag. But before you do make sure that any excess air has been expelled then turn the sealed bag over several times to ensure that the steak is well coated in the marinade. Place the bag on a plate and either leave to marinate at room temperature for 15 minutes or place in the refrigerator for 1 hour. Whilst the meat is marinating in the sauce make sure that you turn the bag over regularly several times.

3. If you have decided to let the steak marinate in the refrigerator remove it 15 minutes before you start cooking to let it come up to room temperature. In fact you should get the barbecue going as you remove the meat from the refrigerator.

4. Whilst you are still waiting for the barbecue to reach the right temperature for cooking the meat to make cooking the onions a lot easier on it thread them on to a metal skewer. Once you have done this set them to one side.

5. Once the meat has now reached room temperature remove from the back and any marinade that remains should be poured into a saucepan and heated up over a high heat. Once it reaches boiling point allow it to continue to boil for 2 minutes before then removing from the heat.

6. Next you need to place the steak and the onions on to the lightly oiled barbecue grill and close the lid. Cook the meat and onions for between 10 and 12 minutes depending on how you like your steak cooked. It is important that you not only turn the steak over regularly whilst it is cooking to ensure that it is cooked evenly throughout but also allows you then to baste it with the remaining marinade.

7. Once the onions and steak are cooked transfer the meat to a cutting board and let it stand for a few minutes. Whilst the meat is standing separate the cooked onion into rings.

8. After resting the steak thinly slice it across the grain and then arrange slices of the onion and steak on top of 4 slices of the sourdough bread that you could have grilled on the barbecue as well before then spooning over some of the juices from the meat.

Now finally place on top of the meat and onions a slice of tomato and some of the arugula before topping of with another slice of bread.

Recipe 11 – Beef Sliders Stuffed With Walnuts and Gorgonzola

These burgers may only be small in size but they deliver on the taste front. Adding of the arugula helps to provide a peppery accent to the rest of the food and although cheese is included these still on contain 249 calories per slider.

Ingredients

500grams Regular Ground Beef
1 Teaspoon Olive Oil
4 Slices Bacon Finely Chopped
25grams Finely Chopped Shallots
25grams Finely Chopped Button Mushrooms
1 Teaspoon Salt
1 Teaspoon Finely Ground Black Pepper
1 Teaspoon Worcestershire Sauce
1 Egg Lightly Beaten
125grams Gorgonzola Divided Into 6 Portions (If you don't like Gorgonzola you can use any other blue cheese instead)
32 Walnut Halves

Instructions

1. Into a frying pan or skillet place the olive oil and then to this add the finely chopped bacon and cook until it has become a golden color then to this add the shallots and cook until they become translucent. Then add to this the mushrooms and continue cooking until all water evaporates from the pan. This should take around 5 minutes to happen.

NB: If you choose not to add bacon to your patties then fry the shallots and mushrooms in 2 teaspoons of olive oil.

2. Once all the above ingredients are cooked transfer them to a bowl and allow to cool down. After the mixture has cooled down you can now add to this the salt and pepper, Worcestershire sauce and egg. Then add to this mixture the ground beef and gently mix together by hand until everything has become incorporated.

3. Now divide the mixture into 16 equal portions and form them into patties. Each one should be about 1 ½ inches thick and 2 ½ inches in diameter. Now into the centre of each patty you tuck a piece of the cheese and 2 walnut halves.

4. Once you have finished creating the patties cover them over and place in the refrigerator whilst you wait for the barbecue to heat up. It is best if you cook them on a medium to high heat and watch them to ensure that you cook them to the way your guests like.

5. As soon as the patties have been cooked the way your guests like serve them immediately in a small dinner roll or between slices of baguette.

Recipe 12 – Lamb Burgers and Fruity Relish

The great thing about making your own burgers is that you will know exactly what is in them. Plus using fresh ingredients ensures that your body is being provided with vital nutrients, minerals and vitamins that it needs.

Ingredients

Burgers
400grams Lean Ground Lamb
1 Carrot Grated
1 Small Onion Finely Chopped
100grams Fresh Whole Wheat Breadcrumbs
1/8 Teaspoon Freshly Grated Nutmeg
2 Teaspoons Fresh Thyme Leaves (If you cannot get fresh thyme leaves use 1 teaspoon of dried thyme leaves instead)
Freshly Ground Pepper To Taste
1 Large Egg Lightly Beaten
2 Tablespoons Extra Virgin Olive Oil

Fruity Relish

1 Orange
100grams Fresh or Frozen Raspberries (Make Sure You Thaw The Frozen Ones Out)
2 Teaspoons Dark Brown Sugar

Instructions

1. In a large bowl place the minced lamb, grated carrot, finely chopped onion, whole wheat breadcrumbs, nutmeg, thyme and pepper. Then mix together roughly with a wooden spoon before then adding the lightly beaten egg. After adding the eggs use your hands to combine all these ingredients together thoroughly.

2. Once you have combined all the above ingredients together divide into four equal amounts and form into patties measuring 10 by 12 inches in diameter. Then put to one side whilst you wait for the barbecue to heat up. Make sure that the patties are covered whilst you are waiting for the barbecue to heat up.

3. As soon as the barbecue has heated up brush each side of the patties with some olive oil and place on the grill which you have set about 6 inches above the heat source. Then cook on each side for about 4 to 5 minutes dependent on just how thick each patty is.

4. Whilst the patties (burgers) are cooking you can now make the relish to go with them. First off remove the peel and pith from the orange using a sharp knife. Make sure that you do this over a bowl so any orange juice that comes out is caught.

5. After removing the pith and peel cut between the membrane and release each segment of the orange. Now roughly chop up each segment and add them to the bowl with the juice in it. Then to this add the raspberries and sugar and lightly crush the fruit together using a fork. Set to one side ready to serve with the burgers.

6. Once the burgers are cooked place each one on to a burger roll, which you have toasted on the barbecue and top each one with a spoonful of the relish you have just made.

Recipe 13 – Chicken Burgers and Tropical Fruit Salsa

Just because you are trying to lose weight it doesn't mean that you have to give up burgers completely. You will find that not only do these burgers contain very little fat but also taste absolutely delicious.

Ingredients

Burgers
500grams Ground Chicken
1 Large Granny Smith Apple Peeled And Shredded
22.5grrams Dry Breadcrumbs

Tropical Fruit Salsa

1 Small Pineapple Cored, Sliced And Chopped
1 Small Mango Peeled And Finely Chopped
1 Small Red Onion Finely Chopped
2 Tablespoons Fresh Finely Chopped Coriander
1 Tablespoon Fresh Lemon Juice
1 Teaspoon Canola Oil

Instructions

1. In a bowl place the cored, sliced and chopped pineapple. Now add to this the mango, red onion, lemon juice, oil and coriander and mix well together. Then set aside for use later.

2. Take the ground chicken, shredded apple and breadcrumbs and place in a bowl and mix well to all ingredients are combined. Once all ingredients have been combined well together now divide into four equal portions and then shape into burgers. Each burger should be about an inch thick. Place these burgers on to a plate and put in to the freezer for 20 minutes. Freezing the burgers will help them to retain their shape when cooking them.

3. Whilst the burgers are in the freezer you can start heating up the barbecue. As soon as the barbecue is ready remove the burgers from the freezer and place them on to the lightly oiled grill and cook until they have turned brown. To check that they are cooked through piece the thickest part of the burger with a skewer or the point of a knife to see if the juices inside run clear.

4. Once the burgers are cooked placed on a whole wheat bun and top with a slice of cheese.

Recipe 14 – Honey Soy Pork Chops

This is a very quick and simple recipe to prepare and cook, but will have your guests asking for more.

Ingredients

4 Boneless Pork Loin Chops
60ml Lemon Juice
60ml Honey
2 Tablespoons Reduced Sodium Soy Sauce
1 Tablespoon Sherry
2 Garlic Cloves Minced

Instructions

1. In a small bowl whisk together the lemon juice, honey, soy sauce, sherry and garlic and then pour half of this in to a resealable bag. As for the remaining mix leave in bowl then cover and place in the refrigerator for use later.

2. In to the resealable bag you now place the pork loin chops and then after closing the bag up turn it over several times to ensure that the chops are well coated in the marinade. Now place the bag in the refrigerator and leave there for 2 to 3 hours.

3. After the marinade time has elapsed remove the pork chops from the refrigerator you should start the barbecue up. After removing the chops from the refrigerator remove them from the bag and place them on a plate to allow them to come up to room temperature.

Any leftover marinade in the bag can now be discarded. It is important that you place the grill about 4 to 6 inches above the heat source as you will want to cook the chops on a medium to high heat.

4. Before you place the chops on the barbecue grill brush some oil over it first to prevent them from sticking. Now cook the chops until they are no longer pink in the middle, which should be about

4 to 5 minutes on each side, making sure that you baste them regularly with the other marinade you put to one side earlier.

If you don't want to cut into the meat to check to see if it is done then insert a meat thermometer into the center of the chop. It is ready when the interior temperature of the meat has reached 145 degrees Fahrenheit.

Recipe 15 – Apple Glazed Pork

We all know how well apple and pork go together and this is one barbecue recipe you will find yourself enjoying time and time again. Each serving provides you with 225 calories and 3.2g of fat. Although a very simple recipe to prepare the meat will need to be allowed to marinade overnight.

Ingredients

6 Boneless Pork Chops
4 Granny Smith Apples Cored And Chopped
1 Can Crushed Pineapple With Juice
120ml Apple Cider Vinegar
32grams Brown Sugar
60ml Dijon Mustard
60ml Water
2 Tablespoons Honey
4 Garlic Cloves Crushed
2 Teaspoons Cayenne Pepper
1 Teaspoon Onion Powder

Instructions

1. Into a large saucepan place the chopped apple, crushed pineapple juice, vinegar, brown sugar, mustard, water, honey, garlic, cayenne pepper and onion powder and bring to the boil over a high heat. Once the ingredients start boiling turn the heat down to medium to low and cover the saucepan. Allow the ingredients inside to simmer for about 15 minutes or until the apples have turned soft. Once the apples have turned soft remove the saucepan from heat and allow the ingredients to cool down to room temperature.

2. As soon as the ingredients in the saucepan have cooled down enough place them in a blender and turn on until a puree is formed.

3. Next take the pork chops and place these into a resealable bag and then pour over them the apple puree you made earlier. Seal the bag and place the bag in the refrigerator and let the chops marinate in the apple puree overnight.

4. When it comes to cooking the chops remove them from the refrigerator just before you start the barbecue up. This will then allow the chops to come up to room temperature and will then be ready for placing on the barbecue once it has heated up.

The grill for the barbecue should not only be lightly oiled but be placed at least 6 inches above the heat source as you will be cooking the chops on a medium heat.

5. After removing the chops from the bag shake of any excess marinade and then discard the rest. Then place the chops on to the barbecue and cook on each side for about 5 minutes.

How long you cook them for will depend on how thick each chop is. The thicker the chop the longer they will need to be cooked for. Chops are ready when they no longer are pink in color inside.

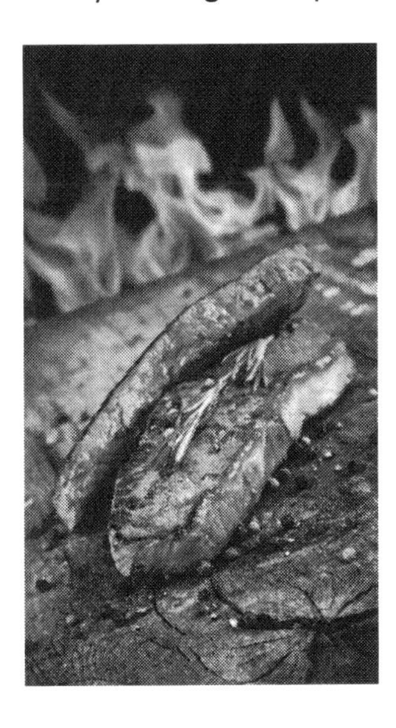

Recipe 16 – Teriyaki Pork Chops With Blueberry Ginger Relish

Each portion of this particular recipe contains only 229 calories and 8g of fat. We recommend you use normal dry sherry rather than cooking sherry, as it doesn't contain so much sodium in it.

Ingredients

4 Bone In Center Cut Pork Chops With Fat Trimmed Off
3 Tablespoons Reduced Sodium Soy Sauce
2 Tablespoons Dry Sherry
2 Garlic Cloves Crushed
1 Teaspoon Brown Sugar
¼ Teaspoon Crushed Red Pepper

Blueberry Ginger Relish

100grams Fresh Blueberries Coarsely Chopped
1 Shallot Chopped
1 Serrano Chilli Seeded And Minced
1 Tablespoon Fresh Cilantro Chopped
1 Tablespoon Lime Juice
1 Teaspoon Fresh Ginger Minced
¼ Teaspoon Salt

Instructions

1. In a bowl whisk together the soy sauce, sherry, garlic, brown sugar and red pepper.

2. Once the marinade is ready place the 4 pork chops into a resealable bag and pour the sauce over them. Seal the bag and then turn it over several times to ensure that the chops have been evenly coated with the marinade. Now place in the refrigerator for at least 2 hours. But to get more of the flavor of the marinade into the chops it is best to leave them in the refrigerator overnight.

3. As for the relish this needs to be prepared 20 minutes before you actually start grilling the chops on the barbecue. To make the relish you simply place the blueberries, ginger, shallot, chilli,

cilantro, salt and lime juice in a bowl and stir well. Once made place to one side ready for serving with the chops after they have cooked.

4. The chops need to be cooked on a high heat on the barbecue so place the lightly oiled grill on which you are placing them about 4 inches above the heat source. Grill each chop for 3 to 5 minutes on each side or until the inside of them is no longer pink.

Once cooked remove from barbecue and place on a clean plate to rest for 5 minutes. After the chops have rested place on further clean plates and serve with some of the relish made earlier.

Recipe 17 – Spanish Pork Burgers

This recipe really does offer a taste of summer. Yet the use of paprika in this recipe helps to give the burgers a slight kick.

Ingredients

450grams Lean Ground Pork
1 Tablespoon Extra Virgin Olive Oil
300grams Spanish Onion Thinly Sliced
¾ Teaspoon Fresh Ground Black Pepper
¼ Teaspoon Salt
1 Tablespoon Finely Chopped Spanish Green Olives
2 Teaspoons Minced Garlic
2 Teaspoons Pimento de la Vera or Hungarian Paprika

Instructions

1. Heat the olive oil in a large frying pan and to this add the onion, ¼ teaspoon of fresh ground black pepper, and salt. Cover the frying pan and cook until the onions have become soft and translucent.

Make sure that you stir the onions occasionally to prevent them from burning. It should take about 10 minutes for the onions to cook. Now divide the onions into two equal portions, as one portion will be used as a topping for the burgers once cooked.

2. First off chop up the other half of the onions and place them in a cool once they have cooled down. Then in to the bowl place the pork, garlic, paprika and olives. Along with the rest of the freshly ground pepper and salt.

Combine all these ingredients together very gently ensuring that everything has been combined together well. Then form the mixture into four equal size burgers. Each one should be about an inch thick. Now place in the freezer to rest whilst you are heating up the barbecue.

3. Once the barbecue has heated up remove the burgers from the freezer and place on the grill, which has been lightly oiled and is 6 inches above the heat source. Cook them on the barbecue for between 10 and 12 minutes or until the inside of the burger is no longer pink in color. Make sure that you turn the burgers over occasionally to prevent them from burning.

4. Just before you remove the burgers from the barbecue place some whole wheat buns on to the grill and toast them lightly. Remove then place the burgers on top and then on top of this place some of the other onions you fried off earlier on top.

Recipe 18 – Grilled Rib Eye Steak with Tomato Salad and Chimichurri Sauce

The sauce that you make to go with this type of steak is a favorite in Argentina and helps to enhance the flavor of the meat further. Each serving contains 257 calories and 13g fat.

Ingredients

Steak
450grams Boneless Rib Eye Steak About 1 Inch Thick Cut Into 4 Portions And Fat Trimmed Off
½ Teaspoon Extra Virgin Olive Oil
¼ Teaspoon Salt
¼ Teaspoon Freshly Ground Black Pepper

Sauce

50grams Fresh Parsley or Cilantro
10grams Fresh Oregano Leaves (Optional)
3 to 6 Garlic Cloves
2 Tablespoons Chopped Onion
120ml Olive Oil
2 Tablespoons Red Wine Vinegar (Optional)
1 Tablespoon Lime Juice (Optional)
Salt and Red Pepper Flakes To Taste

Salad

4 Medium Size Tomatoes Cut Into Wedges
50grams Sweet Onion Thinly Sliced
2 Teaspoons Extra Virgin Olive Oil
1 Tablespoon Distilled White Vinegar
¼ Teaspoon Salt
¼ Teaspoon Freshly Ground Black Pepper

Instructions

1. To make the Chimichurri sauce place the garlic and onion in a blender and mix on pulse until finely chopped. Now to this add the parsley and cilantro and oregano (if using it) and pulse again very briefly again these ingredients are finely chopped.

Now place this mixture into a bowl and add the olive oil, lime juice and vinegar and stir well. You need to add the liquids to the other ingredients in a bowl to ensure that the right texture is achieved. Then season with some salt and the red pepper flakes. Cover and store in the refrigerator ready for use later.

2. Whilst the barbecue is heating up you can now start preparing the salad. Simply place the tomatoes, onion and vinegar into a bowl and stir until the tomatoes and onion are covered in the vinegar. Then sprinkle on some salt and pepper to taste. Again cover this bowl and put to one side ready to use when the steaks are cooked.

3. To cook the steaks make sure that you place the grill as close to the heat source as possible as you want to cook them on a high heat. Just before placing the steaks on the barbecue grill rub them

with the olive oil and season both sides of the steak with salt and pepper. To achieve medium rare steaks cook them on each side for between 3 and 4 minutes.

Allow the steaks to rest for 5 minutes before placing them on to clean plates with some of the tomato salad and a spoonful of the Chimichurri sauce placed on top of the steak.

Recipe 19 – Steak and Potato Kebabs with Creamy Cilantro Sauce

The potatoes you use need to be cooked partially before you put them on to skewers with the steak. If they are not cooked beforehand they will still be hard when the steak is cooked. Serve these kebabs with a fresh green salad or some rice.

Ingredients

Kebabs
600grams Strip Steak Trimmed And Cut Into 1 ½ Inch Pieces
2 Poblano Peppers or 1 Large Green Bell Pepper Cut Into 1 Inch Pieces
1 Large Sweet Onion Cut Into 1 Inch Pieces
8 New Or Baby Red Potatoes
1 Teaspoon Extra Virgin Olive Oil

Sauce

12 ½ grams Fresh Cilantro Leaves Minced
2 Tablespoons Red Wine Vinegar or Cider Vinegar
2 Tablespoons Reduced Fat Sour Cream
1 Small Garlic Clove Minced
1 Teaspoon Chilli Powder
½ Teaspoon Ground Cumin
½ Teaspoon Salt (Divided)

Instructions

1. To make the creamy cilantro sauce combine together the minced cilantro, sour cream, garlic, chilli powder, and cumin and ¼

teaspoon in a small bowl. Now place in the refrigerator ready to use later.

2. Whilst the barbecue is heating up place the potatoes into a container that is microwave safe and cook them on high until they become tender. About 3 to 3 ½ minutes should be sufficient time to cook them in.

3. After cooking the potatoes allow them cool then place them in a bowl with the steak and pepper pieces and pour over the oil and some salt. Then toss to make sure that all ingredients are coated in the oil.

4. Now thread the steak, potatoes, peppers and onions on to skewers in an alternate pattern. By now the barbecue should have heated up so apply a light coating of oil to the grill and place the kebabs on it.

Cook for about 6 minutes turning once or twice whilst they are cooking. When the kebabs are cooked to the way you or your guests like remove from barbecue place on clean plates and add a spoonful of sauce beside them.

Recipe 20 – Grilled Filet Mignon with Herb Butter and Texas Toasts

This very simple dish tastes very luxurious because of the herb butter. Even when you eat it with the toast made from whole grain bread this actual recipe only contains 303 calories and 14 grams of fat.

Ingredients

450grams Steak Filet Mignon Cut Into 4 Portions That Are 1 ½ Inches Thick And With The Fat Trimmed Off
1 Tablespoon Slightly Softened Butter
3 Teaspoons Extra Virgin Olive Oil (Divided)
1 Tablespoon Fresh Chives Or Shallots Minced
1 Tablespoon Capers Rinsed And Chopped
3 Teaspoons Fresh Marjoram Or Oregano Minced (Divided)
1 Teaspoon Freshly Grated Lemon Zest (Divided)

1 Teaspoon Lemon Juice
¾ Teaspoon Salt (Divided)
½ Teaspoon Freshly Ground Black Pepper (Divided)
1 Tablespoon Fresh Rosemary Minced
2 Garlic Cloves (1 Minced And 1 Peeled And Halved)
4 Slices Whole Grain Bread
4 Cups Fresh Watercress Trimmed And Chopped

Instructions

1. In a small bowl mash together the softened butter with the back of a spoon and to this stir in 2 teaspoons of the oil until both ingredients are well combined. Now add to this the shallots or chives along with the capers a teaspoon of marjoram or oregano, ½ teaspoon of lemon zest, the lemon juice, ½ teaspoon of salt and ¼ teaspoon of black pepper. Once all these ingredients have been mixed together thoroughly cover the bowl and place in the freezer to chill.

2. Next in another bowl mix together the rest of the oil (1 teaspoon), 2 teaspoons of marjoram or oregano, ½ teaspoon of lemon zest, ¼ teaspoon of salt and pepper, the rosemary and minced garlic. Take this mixture after thoroughly combined and rub into both sides of the steaks. As for the other garlic that has been cut half you rub this over both sides of the bread.

3. Once the barbecue is ready you can now place the steaks on the grill that should be around 6 inches above the heat source. Cook each steak for between 3 and 5 minutes on each side so that they become medium rare. During the last minute of cooking the steak place the bread on the grill and toast each side for 30 seconds.

4. Remove the steaks from the barbecue and let them rest whilst you prepare the plates on which they are to be served. Whilst the steaks are resting spread some of the herb butter over the top. First place a handful of watercress on to each plate and on top of this place a piece of the toast before then topping off with the steak.

Chapter 2 – Healthy Seafood Recipes for the Barbecue

Recipe 1 – Grilled Oyster Shooters

This is a very quick and simple meal not only to prepare but also to cook. Each oyster contains only 32 calories and 0.2g fat.

Ingredients

8 Fresh Oysters In Shells
80ml Fresh Lemon Juice
3 Tablespoons Worcestershire Sauce
Hot Pepper Sauce To Taste
Salt To Taste

Instructions

1. Preheat your barbecue and place the grill 4 inches above the heat source as you will want to cook the oysters on a high heat.

2. As soon as the barbecue as heated up place the unopened oysters on to the grill and cook until they start to open. This should take around 5 to 10 minutes. You will know when they have opened up, as you will hear a sizzling sound as some of the juices form inside the oysters fall on to the hot coals.

3. You now remove the oysters from the grill and pry off the top shell. It may be a good idea to wear some good quality kitchen gloves to do this in order to protect your hands from the heat. Once the top shell is removed take a sharp knife and slide it between the oyster and the bottom part of the shell to disconnect it.

4. After disconnecting the oyster from the shell let it remain in it and then top it off with 2 teaspoons of lemon juice a teaspoon of Worcestershire sauce and some hot pepper sauce and salt to taste.

Recipe 2 - Grilled Fish Tacos with Chipotle Lime Dressing

Don't be too surprised if your guests keep asking for more of these because they taste so delicious.

Ingredients

450grams Tilapia Fillet Cut Into Chunks

Marinade

60ml Extra Virgin Olive Oil
2 Tablespoons Distilled Wine Vinegar
2 Tablespoons Fresh Lime Juice
2 Teaspoons Fresh Lime Zest
1 ½ Teaspoons Honey
2 Garlic Cloves Minced
½ Teaspoon Cumin
½ Teaspoon Chilli Powder
1 Teaspoon Seafood Seasoning
½ Teaspoon Freshly Ground Black Pepper
1 Teaspoon Hot Pepper Sauce To Taste

Dressing

220ml Light Sour Cream
120ml Adobo Sauce From Chipotle Peppers
2 Tablespoons Fresh Lime Juice
2 Teaspoons Fresh Lime Zest
¼ Teaspoon Cumin
¼ Teaspoon Chilli Powder
½ Teaspoon Seafood Seasoning
Salt And Freshly Ground Black Pepper To Taste

Tacos

1 Packet Tortillas
3 Ripe Tomatoes Seeded And Diced
1 Bunch Fresh Cilantro Chopped
1 Small Cabbage Head Cored And Shredded
2 Limes Cut In To Wedges

Instructions

1. In a bowl you need to make the marinade. To do this whisk together the olive oil, wine vinegar, lime juice and zest, honey, minced garlic, cumin, chilli powder, seafood seasoning, black pepper and hot sauce until thoroughly combined.

2. Next place the chunks of fish into a shallow dish and over this pour the marinade you have just made. Cover the dish and place in the refrigerator for 6 to 8 hours.

3. Whilst the fish is marinating you can start to make the dressing, which you will serve the fish with after it has been cooked. To make the dressing in to a bowl place the adobo sauce and sour cream then very gently stir into this the lime juice and zest along with the cumin, chilli powder, seafood seasoning and salt and pepper to taste. Now cover over and place in the refrigerator until it is needed.

4. After removing the fish from the refrigerator you should now get the barbecue heated up and set the grill which will need to be oiled before cooking starts to 4 inches above the heat source. This is because you will be cooking the fish on a high heat.

5. As soon as the barbecue is hot enough remove the fish from the marinade and discard any that is left over. It is important that before you place the fish chunks on the barbecue that you drain of any excess and then grill the fish until it flakes easily with a fork. Each piece of fish should only need about 9 minutes on the barbecue with them being turned over once.

6. Once the fish is cooked assembly of the tacos can begin. To assemble the tacos place pieces of the cooked fish on to the center of a warm tortilla and on top of these place some of the diced tomatoes, chopped cilantro and shredded cabbage then drizzle with the dressing you made earlier. Now roll the tortillas up and serve them to your guests with a lime wedge.

Recipe 3 – Grilled Tuna with Zucchini Pasta and Artichoke Sauce

This really is a healthy way to have a pasta like side order with your grilled tuna and means you are cutting down on your carbs. If you can afford to buy tuna steaks that have been caught either using a hook and line or poll and line.

Ingredients

4 Tuna Steaks Weighing 170grams Each
Salt and Freshly Ground Black Pepper To Taste
Oil For Cooking

Zucchini Pasta

950grams Green And Gold Zucchini
2 Teaspoons Salt

Artichoke Sauce

450grams Tomatoes Peeled, Seeded And Diced
1 Medium Sized Onion Diced
3 Garlic Cloves Minced
1 Teaspoon Salt
250ml Marinated Baby Artichokes Diced
1-2 Teaspoons Freshly Minced Hot Or Mild Chilli Pepper To Taste
65ml Fresh Basil Chopped
Freshly Ground Black Pepper To Taste

Black Olive Tapenade

250ml Pitted Kalamata Olives (Or Black Olives You Like)
1 Garlic Cloves Minced
1 Tablespoon Capers
65ml Fresh Basil Leaves Chopped
65ml Fresh Flat Leaf Parsley Chopped
Pinch Crushed Red Pepper Flakes
1 Tablespoon Red Or White Wine Vinegar
125ml Extra Virgin Olive Oil
Some Salt And Freshly Ground Black Pepper To Taste

Instructions

1. To make the tapenade in a bowl combine together the olives, garlic, capers, basil, parsley, red pepper flakes, wine vinegar and olive oil. Then add some salt and pepper to taste. Once all these have been combined well together cover and set to one side. Do not place in the refrigerator.

2. Now move on to making the zucchini pasta. To do this take a sharp knife and cut off the tops and bottoms of each and then cut them in half lengthwise. Now take a cheese slice and very slowly slice down each cut half of the zucchini to make thin ribbons.

Once you have sliced all the zucchini up place in a colander and toss them in some salt and leave to sit for 15 minutes when they should have an al dente feel to them. In fact just before you start to make the pasta you should get the barbecue started.

3. Whilst the pasta is resting you can now make the sauce to go with it. In a heavy bottom pan place the oil, onion, garlic and sauce and cook until the onions have become translucent in color around 5 to 7 minutes. Then to this add the crushed tomatoes and cook on a low heat for a further 30 minutes. After this time now add the artichokes, chilli pepper and basil and let cook for another 10 minutes on a low heat. Before placing to one side to cool add some freshly ground black pepper to taste.

4. To cook the tuna steaks you must remove them from the refrigerator 15 minutes before and grill over a medium to high heat. Cook each steak for between 4 to 6 minutes making sure that you turn them half way through the cooking time. You will know when the tuna is ready because the middle should still be pink but the edges will flake easily.

5. Once the tuna steaks are cooked serve them on the zucchini that has been tossed in the sauce you made earlier. Then on top of the tuna place a spoonful of the tapenade.

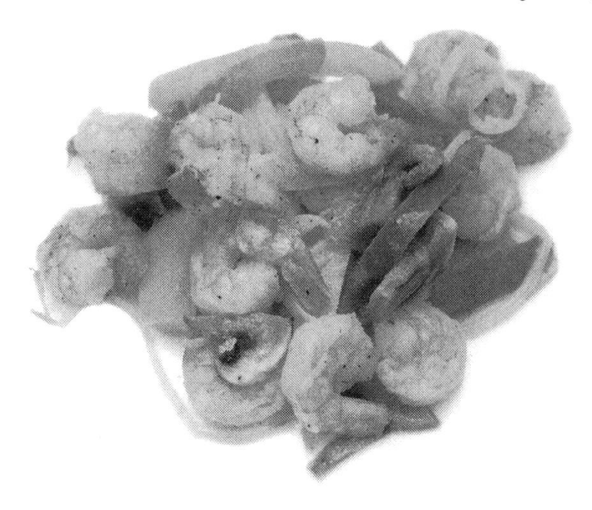

Recipe 4 – Thai Spiced Barbecue Shrimp

This is an extremely healthy meal to serve at any barbecue. Each serving contains only 73 calories and 1g fat.

Ingredients

450grams Medium Sized Shrimps Deveined And Peeled
3 Tablespoons Fresh Lemon Juice
1 Tablespoon Soy Sauce
1 Tablespoon Dijon Mustard
2 Garlic Cloves Minced
1 Tablespoon Brown Sugar
2 Teaspoons Curry Paste

Instructions

1. Into either a shallow dish or resealable bag mix together the lemon juice, soy sauce, mustard, garlic, sugar and curry paste and to this then add the shrimps. Now either cover the dish or seal the bag up and place in the refrigerator to allow the shrimps to marinate in the sauce for 1 hour.

2. Whilst the shrimps are marinating in the refrigerator this would be a good time to get the barbecue started. It is important that you place the grill, which needs to be oiled before the shrimps are

placed on it 4 inches above the heat source, as the shrimps need to be cooked on a high heat.

3. To cook the shrimps thread them first on to some skewers if you intend to use wooden ones then these should have been soaked in water for at least 30 minutes to prevent them from burning.

However if you have a grill basket then place them inside this instead as it makes handling them much easier. Any leftover marinade should be transferred to a saucepan and boiled for a few minutes.

4. To cook the shrimps they should be grilled on each side for 3 minutes or until they turn opaque. Make sure that whilst they are cooking that you baste them regularly with the left over marinade in the saucepan.

Recipe 5 – Fish Steaks with Grilled Fennel, Red Peppers and Onions

The grilled fennel, red peppers and onions are not only extremely beneficial to your health but also help to bring out the flavor of the fish even more. Although each serving contains 349 calories and 16g fat none of the fat in this recipe is of the saturated kind.

Ingredients

4 x 170gram Cod Steaks That Is 1 Inch Thick
60ml Extra Virgin Olive Oil
2 Tablespoons Fresh Lemon Juice
1 Tablespoon Freshly Chopped Oregano
1 ½ Teaspoons Freshly Chopped Rosemary
½ Teaspoon Coarse Sea Salt
½ Teaspoon Freshly Ground Black Pepper
1 Garlic Clove
2 Small Fennel Bulbs Tops Removed Bulbs Quartered Through Root End
2 Red Bell Peppers Seeded And Quartered
2 Sweet Onions Cut Into ½ Inch Thick Slices
Lemon Wedges

Instructions

1. In a bowl combine together the olive oil, lemon juice, oregano, rosemary, salt, black pepper and garlic. Now set to one side.

2. Next heat up the barbecue and place the grill 4 to 6 inches above the heat source, as you will want to cook the fish steaks on a medium to high heat.

Once the barbecue has heated up, brush the grill with some oil and then brush the vegetables with the mixture you made earlier and place on the grill. Cook until they are lightly charred and are just starting to go soft.

This should take around 12 minutes and you should make sure that during the cooking time you turn the vegetables over regularly. Once the vegetables are cooked remove from barbecue place on a plate and cover to keep them warm.

3. After removing the vegetables from the grill brush it again with some oil and then brush the fish steaks with some more of the sauce you made earlier. Grill each one for 10 minutes or until the fish turns opaque. It is important whilst cooking the fist you turn them over once to ensure that the steaks are cooked right through.

4. Once the fish steaks are cooked place each on a plate on top of some of the vegetables and then drizzle some more extra virgin olive oil over the top. Serve with lemon wedges.

Recipe 6 – Grilled Salmon with Dill Pickle Butter

The great about cooking salmon on a barbecue is that you don't need to worry about whether it is cooked all the way through or not, as it can be served rare to medium to your guests.

Ingredients

4 x 170gram Salmon Fillets With Skin
4 Tablespoons Unsalted Butter Softened
60grams Dill Pickles Finely Diced
1 Teaspoon Tarragon Minced

½ Teaspoon Dijon Mustard
Salt And Freshly Ground Black Pepper To Taste
Extra Virgin Olive Oil For Rubbing

Instructions

1. Light the barbecue. Whilst the barbecue is heating up you can now make the dill pickle butter. To make the butter in a bowl blend the butter with the diced dill pickles, tarragon and mustard. Then add some salt and pepper to taste. Now place in the refrigerator until needed later.

2. As soon as the barbecue has heated up rub the salmon fillets with olive oil and sprinkle over them salt and pepper. Grill the fillets on a moderately high heat with the skin side down first. Cook on this side of the salmon fillet until the skin has become crisp and lightly charred. This should only take around 3 minutes then turn the fillets over using a metal spatula and cook for another 4 minutes or until the inside of the salmon is barely done.

3. As soon as the salmon is cooked remove from grill place on clean plates and top with a spoonful of the dill pickle butter you made earlier then serve to your guests with some fresh new potatoes and a crisp green salad.

Recipe 7 – Grilled Scallops with Prosciutto

The saltiness of the Italian dried ham (Prosciutto) combines extremely well with the scallops. Each skewer contains 315 calories and 20g of fat of which 6g is saturated.

Ingredients

12 Fresh King Scallops With Corals
16 Thin Slices Prosciutto
Freshly Ground Black Pepper To Taste

Marinade

2 Large Garlic Cloves Crushed
Few Sprigs Of Fresh Basil, Parsley And Coriander

½ Lemon
3 Tablespoons Virgin Olive Oil

Instructions

1. First rinse and dry the scallops then separate the corals from them and place in a bowl.

2. Next make the marinade. To do this place the crushed garlic cloves in a bowl and then add to it some basil, parsley and coriander which has been chopped. Keep a few sprigs of basil to one side, as you will be using this as a garnish later. Now into the bowl squeeze the juice of the lemon and the olive oil and stir until well combined. Leave to marinate at room temperature for 15 minutes. In fact just before you start making the marinade you should get the barbecue started.

3. Once the barbecue is heated up and you have set the grill 4 inches above the heat source you can start preparing the scallops and prosciutto for cooking. First take one slice of the prosciutto and gather it up so it forms a ruffle then thread this on to a metal skewer. Then thread on one of the scallops followed by one of the corals. Do this three more times on four skewers.

4. Once the skewers ready lay them across the grill of the barbecue, which has been lightly oiled, and then brush over some of the marinade. Grill each skewer for 5 minutes making sure that you turn them over after 2 ½ minutes and baste them regularly with the marinade you made earlier. They are ready to serve when the prosciutto is crisp and the scallops are just cooked.

5. After placing on to clean plates spoon over a little more of the marinade and serve to your guests topped off with some sprigs of basil.

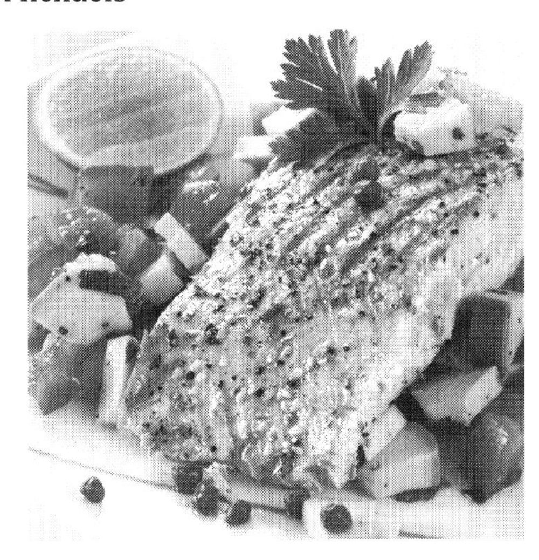

Recipe 8 – Grilled Salmon with Zucchini and Red Pepper Sauce

The Spanish inspired sauce that you serve with this fish helps to jazz it up a great deal. But not only does it go great with all kinds of fish but is also great when served with poultry or vegetables. The addition of paprika to the sauce helps to enhance the flavors of the grill even more. Each serving contains just 280 calories and 13g fat.

Ingredients

567grams Salmon Fillet Cut Into Four Equal Size Portions
78grams Sliced Almonds Toasted
60grams Jarred Roasted Red Peppers Chopped
60grams Cherry Tomatoes Halved
1 Garlic Clove
1 Tablespoon Extra Virgin Olive Oil
1 Teaspoon Smoked Paprika
¾ Teaspoon Salt (Divided)
½ Teaspoon Freshly Ground Black Pepper (Divided)
2 Medium Zucchini Cut In Half Lengthwise
Canola or Olive Oil For Cooking
1 Tablespoon Fresh Parsley Chopped To Garnish

Instructions

1. Preheat the barbecue placing the grill 6 inches above the heat source, as you will be cooking the salmon on a medium heat.

2. Now in to a food processor place the toasted almonds, peppers, tomatoes, garlic, olive oil, paprika, ¼ teaspoon salt and black pepper. Blend until a smooth paste is formed then set to one side.

3. Next coat both the salmon and the zucchini on both sides with canola or olive oil and sprinkle over them the remaining salt and pepper. Then place on the grill. Turn each fish and zucchini at least once during the cooking time. Each side of the salmon and zucchini should be cooked for around 3 minutes. The salmon will be just cooked through after 6 minutes whilst the zucchini will be soft and brown.

3. Now transfer the zucchini to a clean chopping board and allow to cool for a little while. As soon as the zucchini can be handled slice each one into ½ inch pieces and place in bowl and add to this some of the sauce made earlier.

Toss very gently ensuring that all pieces of the zucchini are coated in the sauce then transfer it to 4 plates. Now top of the piles of zucchini with the salmon fillets and then top off with the rest of the sauce before then garnishing with parsley.

Recipe 9 – Grilled Halibut with Tomato Basil Sauce

If you have seasoned the sauce properly it really helps to dress up what can be quite a boring fish. Serving 1 halibut fillet with 3 tablespoons of sauce only contains 203 calories and 5g fat of which 1g is saturated fat.

Ingredients

2 x 170gram Halibut Fillets
1 Tablespoon Lemon Juice
1 ½ Teaspoons Fresh Rosemary Minced or ½ Teaspoon Dried Rosemary Crushed
1 ½ Teaspoons Olive Oil
¼ Teaspoon Salt
Dash Freshly Ground Black Pepper

60grams Tomatoes Seeded And Diced
1 Tablespoon Fresh Basil Minced or 1 Teaspoon Dried Basil
1 Tablespoon Green Onion Chopped
1 ½ Teaspoons Red Wine Vinegar
¼ Teaspoon Grated Orange Peel

Instructions

1. Into a large resealable bag combine together the lemon juice, rosemary, olive oil, slat and pepper and then to this add the halibut fillets. After sealing the bag turn it over to ensure that the fish fillets are fully covered in the marinade and place in the refrigerator for an hour.

2. About 15 minutes before you remove the fish fillets from the refrigerator you should now get the barbecue started so by the time the fish has returned to room temperature it is ready for cooking on.

3. Once the barbecue is ready for cooking on with the grill placed 6 inches above the heat source lightly oil it and then remove the fish from the marinade. Make sure that you drain the fish well before placing on to the barbecue grill and any marinade left over can now be discarded.

After placing the fish on the grill put the lid down and leave to cook for 4 to 5 minutes. Now raise the lid turn the fish fillets over and cook for a further 4 to 5 minutes or until the fish flakes easily using a fork.

4. Whilst the fish is cooking into a small saucepan place the tomatoes, basil, green onion, red wine vinegar and orange peel and cook over a medium heat until they are heated through.

5. Place the cooked fish on to clean plates and drizzle over them some of the sauce you have just made in the saucepan.

Recipe 10 – Grilled Lobster Rolls

Although lobster is considered quite a rich type of fish it is still extremely healthy for you. This particular recipe contains 310 calories per serving along with 8g fat.

Ingredients

2 x 283 gram Fresh Lobster Tails
(However Frozen Ones Can Be Used But Need To Be Completely Thawed Before They Are Cooked)
2 Teaspoons Extra Virgin Olive Oil
236grams Snow Peas Trimmed
60grams Celery Minced
60grams Reduced Fat Mayonnaise
1 Tablespoon Lemon Juice
2 Teaspoons Lemon Juice
1 Tablespoon Shallot Minced
2 Teaspoons Dijon Mustard
1 Teaspoon Fresh Tarragon Chopped
½ Teaspoon Freshly Ground Black Pepper
1/8 Teaspoon Salt To Taste
¼ Teaspoon Garlic Powder

Instructions

1. Get the barbecue started placing the grill just 4 inches above the heat source, as you will be cooking the lobster tails on a high heat.

2. Take each lobster tail and place on a chopping board with the soft side facing up wards and cut each one in half lengthwise through the shell using some kitchen shears. Now run your fingers inside the shell to help loosen the meat away from the sides and then brush it with oil.

3. Now take the lobster tails and place on the grill cut side down and cook until the meat has become lightly charred and the shell has started to turn read. This should take around 5 or 6 minutes and then continue to cook the lobster tails until the meat has become opaque and the shell is completely red which should take

a further 2 to 4 minutes dependent on the size of each lobster tail. Now transfer the lobster tails to a chopping board.

4. Whilst the lobster tails are cooling bring a small pan of water to the boil and into this put the snow peas and cook until they turn bright green. Drain and then refresh them using some cold water and slice them very thinly.

5. As soon as the lobster tails are cool enough to handle remove the meat from inside and chop coarsely. Then set to one side.

6. Now into a bowl place the celery reduced fat mayonnaise, lemon juice, shallot, Dijon mustard, tarragon, pepper, salt and garlic powder and mix well together. Then to this add the meat from the lobster tails along with the thinly cut snow peas and stir well. Now you can either place the salad you have just made onto toasted whole wheat rolls or serve it back inside the shell of the lobster tails.

Recipe 11 – Tuna Steaks with Salsa

The salsa you serve with the Tuna steaks help to bring out some amazing flavors in the fish after it has been cooked on the barbecue. This is a very healthy option to serve your guests especially those on a diet as each serving contains only 81 calories and 1g fat.

Ingredients

4 x 170gram Tuna Steaks
240grams Carrots Shredded
177grams Fresh Mango Peeled And Chopped
2 Tablespoons Fresh Lime Juice
1 Tablespoon Chives Minced
¼ Teaspoon Salt Divided
¼ Teaspoon Freshly Ground Black Pepper Divided
1/8 Teaspoon Ground Coriander
1/8 Teaspoon Ground Cumin

Instructions

1. To make the salsa in a bowl place the carrots, mango, lime juice, chives, 1/8 teaspoon salt and pepper, coriander and cumin. Mix well together then set to one side.

2. Now whilst the barbecue is heating up you can prepare the tuna steaks for cooking. Simply sprinkle the remaining salt and pepper over them on both sides and set to one side whilst you wait for the barbecue to get hot.

3. As soon as the barbecue has heated up lightly brush some oil over the grill and then place the tuna steaks on to it. Cook them on a medium heat so the grill should be 6 inches above the heat source for 5 to 7 minutes on each side. When you slice the steak open the inside should still be slightly pink in the center.

4. Place the tuna steaks on to 4 plates and beside them serve a couple of spoonful's of the salsa you made earlier then serve to your guests along with a fresh green salad.

Recipe 12 – Hanoi Style Tuna Patty Salad

This particular recipe exemplifies the Vietnamese peoples attitude towards eating healthily. Each serving contains 359 calories and 1g fat.

Ingredients

Tuna Patties

567grams Tuna Steaks
60grams Green Onions (Scallions) Finely Chopped
3 Tablespoons Red Onion Finely Chopped
1 Tablespoon Fresh Ginger Minced
2 Teaspoons Fish Sauce
1 Teaspoon Reduced Sodium Soy Sauce
1 Teaspoon Brown Sugar
½ Teaspoon Freshly Ground Black Pepper

Salad & Dressing

120ml Water

3 Tablespoons Fish Sauce
2 Tablespoons Granulated Sugar
2 Tablespoons Rice Vinegar or Cider Vinegar
2 Tablespoons Fresh Lime Juice
1 Tablespoon Fresh Ginger Minced
1 Small Garlic Clove
340grams Thin Rice Noodles
1420grams Romaine Lettuce Shredded
475grams Mung Bean Sprouts

Instructions

1. The tuna steaks and with a sharp knife chop it into slices using quick even straight up and down motions. Then continue to chop until you have pieces that are roughly ¼ inch in size.

2. Now take the pieces of tuna place them in a bowl and add to them the onions, ginger, fish sauce, soy sauce, brown sugar and pepper and gently combine them together. Now cover the bowl over and refrigerator whilst you prepare the rest of the salad. However if you would like the tuna to take even more of the flavors of the other ingredients then it is a good idea to leave it in the refrigerator overnight.

3. Next you need to make the salad to do this mix the water with the fish sauce, sugar, vinegar, lime juice, ginger and garlic and stir until all the sugar is dissolved. Now take out around 60ml of this mixture, as you will use it later.

4. In a large saucepan bring some water to boiling point then add the rice noodles. Make sure that you stir them well to help separate them and boil until they have become soft but are still resilient about 2 to 5 minutes should be long enough. Drain the noodles then rinse under cold running water then drain well before then transferring to a bowl and toss them in 2 tablespoons of the dressing you reserved earlier.

5. Now in another bowl place the lettuce and bean sprouts and pour over the rest of the salad dressing and toss until all items are coated. Now divide the mixture between 6 shallow serving bowls and then top with the noodles.

6. Whilst the barbecue is heating up remove the tuna from the refrigerator and form it into 6 equal size patties. Place inside a fish basket that you have brushed with oil and then brush the grill of the barbecue with oil before then placing the fish basket with the patties inside on it to cook. Cook until the patties become firm to the touch about 2 to 3 minutes on each side.

7. Once the tuna patties are cooked remove from grill and place one on top of the salad you made earlier and serve to your guests.

Recipe 13 – Shrimp Po' Boy

It is best to use bread that is soft on the inside and crusty on the outside to serve this particular meal on. To really make this dish healthy serve the Shrimp Po' Boy on whole wheat bread. Each serving of this dish is made up of 322 calories and 10g fat.

Ingredients

450grams Shrimps Peeled And Deveined
470grams Red Cabbage Finely Shredded
2 Tablespoons Dill Pickle Relish
2 Tablespoons Reduced Fat Mayonnaise
2 Tablespoons Non Fat Plain Yogurt
4 Teaspoons Canola Oil Divided
1 Teaspoon Chilli Powder
½ Teaspoon Paprika
¼ Teaspoon Freshly Ground Black Pepper

To Serve

4 Whole Wheat Rolls Or Small Baguettes
4 Tomatoes Sliced
60grams Red Onion Thinly Sliced

Instructions

1. Preheat the barbecue to a medium to high heat.

2. In a bowl combine together the shredded cabbage, dill relish, mayonnaise and yogurt. Now set to one side (place in the refrigerator).

3. Into a bowl place two teaspoons of oil along with the chilli powder, paprika and pepper and to this add the shrimps. Then toss very gently to ensure that the shrimps are well coated in the mixture. Again set to one side.

4. Now take the bread rolls and cut in half and then brush the inside of them with some water and then some oil.

5. Place the shrimps into a fish basket making sure that they are spread out evenly over the surface and place them on to the grill. Cook until the shrimps have turned pink in color that should take about 3 minutes. Make sure that you turn them over once to prevent the shrimps from burning.

6. Just before you remove the shrimps from the barbecue you should take the bread rolls and place these on to the grill making sure that only allow them to toast for 30 seconds on each side.

7. Remove the bread rolls from the grill place on to plates and on to them place slices of tomato and onion and spread along the middle some of the cabbage before then topping off with shrimps. Then serve to your guests.

Recipe 14 – Grilled Garlic Shrimp

Although these grilled shrimps taste wonderful on their own they taste just as great when served with pasta, salad or fajitas. Each serving contains 212 calories and 14.5g of fat.

Ingredients

450grams Large Shrimps Peeled And Deveined
4 Garlic Cloves
60ml Olive Oil
¼ Teaspoon Freshly Ground Black Pepper
Salt to Taste

Wooden Skewers Soaked In Water

Instructions

1. Whilst the barbecue is heating up you can now prepare the garlic marinate for the shrimps. On a chopping board cut up the garlic cloves then sprinkle on some salt. Now with the back of a knife smash the garlic until it forms a paste. Once you have done this place the garlic paste into a frying pan (skillet) with the oil and cook until it has turned brown, which should be about 5 minutes. Now remove this from the heat.

2. Next on to each skewer thread 5 large shrimps and then season with salt and pepper. Then brush one side of the shrimps with the garlic infused oil and place them on to the grill of the barbecue and brush with more of the garlic oil.

3. Cook on the first side for 4 minutes before then turning them over, making sure that you brush them with more of the oil before placing them back down on the grill and cook on this side for a further 4 minutes. Once the shrimps have turned opaque remove from heat and serve.

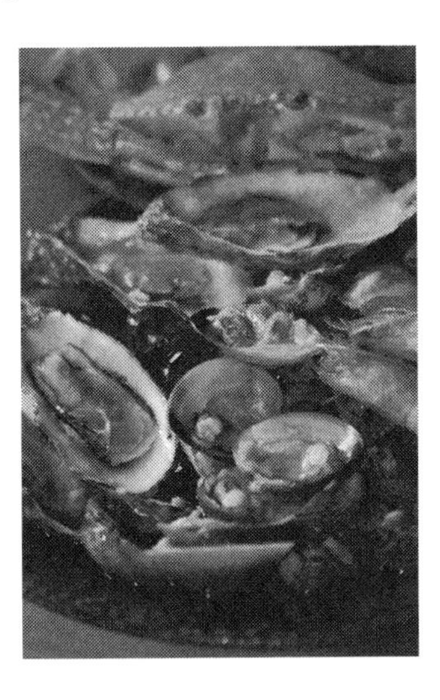

Recipe 15 – Grilled Mussels and Curry Butter

This is an absolutely delicious recipe and can be served either as an appetizer or as a main course. Serve with crusty bread as an appetizer or with a fresh green salad as a main. Each serving contains 299 calories and 14.1g of fat.

Ingredients

907grams Mussels Scrubbed And Debearded
3 Tablespoons Butter Softened
2 Garlic Cloves Pressed
1 Teaspoon Curry Powder
½ Teaspoon Ground Cumin
1/8 Teaspoon Salt
236grams Red Bell Pepper Chopped
60grams Fresh Parsley Chopped
1 Lime Thinly Sliced
1 Lime Cut Into 4 Wedges

Instructions

1. Start up the barbecue and place the grill 6 inches above the heat source, as you want to cook the mussels on a medium heat.

2. Now in a bowl place the softened butter, pressed garlic, curry powder, cumin and slat and whisk together.

3. Take four large pieces of aluminum foil and divide the mussels into four equal amounts and place each amount on to a piece of the foil. Now dot each mussel with the curry butter and then sprinkle over them the chopped red bell pepper and parsley. Then on top of this place a slice of lime. Wrap the foil tightly around the mussels and other ingredients and place the packets on to the grill, which has been lightly oiled.

4. Leave the packets on the barbecue for about 5 to 10 minutes or until the mussels have opened. If you notice that no mussels have opened after this time simply discard them.

5. Now transfer the open mussels to four individual bowls and garnish with a lime wedge before serving to your guests.

Recipe 16 – Orange Scented Grilled Lobster Tails

You may find that the second time you make this recipe that you will need to make double the amount of marinade as your guests will enjoy it so much. Each serving contains 261 calories and 13.1g of fat.

Ingredients

4 x 170grams Lobster Tails
170grams Butter
2 Tablespoons Lemon Juice
1 Tablespoon Grated Orange Zest
1/8 Teaspoon Ground Ginger
1/8 Teaspoon Chilli Powder
1/8 Teaspoon Aromatic Bitters

Instructions

1. Preheat the barbecue and place the grill which should be lightly oiled before the lobster tails are placed on it 6 inches above the heat source. This is because you want to cook the lobster tails on a medium heat.

2. Whilst the barbecue is heating up place the butter in a saucepan on a medium heat and melt. Then stir into it the lemon juice, orange zest, ginger, chilli powder and aromatic bitters. Simmer gently for 2 minutes then set to one side.

3. Cut away the membrane on the underside of each lobster tail and then insert a metal skewer into them. Doing this will prevent the tail from curling as the lobster cooks.

4. Place the lobster tails on to the grill shell side up and cook for 10 minutes, then turn the tails over. After you turn the tails over now spoon over some of the sauce and cook until the meat in the tails is no longer translucent in the middle. 10 more minutes should suffice.

5. Remove the lobster tails from the barbecue and place on plates with a fresh green crispy salad and some crusty whole wheat or granary bread.

Recipe 17 – Grilled Sweet And Sour Scallops

The scallops should first of all be marinated in rice wine and fresh ginger before then being basted in a sweet soy sauce as they cook. This will provide you with very flavorsome Asian styled grilled scallops.

Ingredients

680grams Sea Scallops Drained
60ml Rice Wine
1 Tablespoon Fresh Ginger Grated
60grams Brown Sugar
60ml Tomato Ketchup
60ml Chicken Broth
2 Tablespoons Rice Vinegar
2 Tablespoons Soy Sauce
1 Teaspoon Cornstarch
1 Teaspoon Sesame Oil
2 Garlic Cloves Minced
¼ to ½ Teaspoon Ground Red Pepper (Optional)

Instructions

1. In a small bowl stir together the 60ml rice wine and grated ginger.

2. Place the scallops into a shallow dish and pour over the mixture you have just made and cover. Now place in the refrigerator and leave the scallops to marinate in sauce for 30 minutes. Whilst the scallops are marinating places wooden skewers in water and leave them to soak.

3. Next you need to make the Sweet and Sour sauce that you will baste the scallops in when cooking. To do this put the sugar, ketchup, chicken broth, rice vinegar, soy sauce, corn-starch, sesame oil and garlic into a saucepan and heat up the ingredients

over a medium heat bringing to the boil. If you want you can also add the ground red pepper to give your sauce a little kick. Boil for 1 minute, stirring constantly then remove from heat and set to one side for use later.

4. 15 minutes before you are due to remove the scallops from the refrigerator get the barbecue going and put the grill 6 inches above the heat source.

5. Remove scallops from refrigerator and thread them on to the skewers. Make sure that you leave a gap of ½ inch between each scallop on the skewers. Any marinade that is left over in the dish can be discarded now.

6. Place the scallops on to the grill, which you have lightly oiled first, and close the lid. Cook for 2 to 3 minutes on each side.

7. Once the scallops are cooked brush first with some of the sauce you made earlier and then place any remaining sauce in a bowl, which your guests can then help themselves to if they want more. Serve the scallops with plain rice and garnish with some freshly chopped parsley and strips of green onion.

Recipe 18 – Grilled Diver Scallops On Rosemary

To make turning the scallops over easier use two rosemary sprigs as skewers. Plus by using the rosemary you are adding more of this wonderful herbs flavor to the scallops.

Ingredients

12 Large Sea Scallops
1 Tablespoon Olive Oil
1 Teaspoon Fresh Rosemary Finely Chopped
1/8 Teaspoon Salt
1/8 Teaspoon Freshly Ground Black Pepper
8 x 12 Inch Fresh Sprigs Of Rosemary

Instructions

1. In a bowl combine together the olive oil, fresh rosemary, salt and black pepper. Then to this mixture add the scallops making sure that they are covered well before covering the bowl and placing them scallops in the refrigerator to marinate in the sauce for 30 minutes.

2. Whilst the scallops are in the refrigerator now you should get the barbecue going so by the time you are ready to cook the scallops the required temperature to cook them at has been reached.

3. Next take the 8 sprigs of rosemary and remove 6 inches of the leaves off one end of each. Now place these sprigs into a shallow dish full of water and leave them to soak in it for 20 minutes. Doing this will prevent the rosemary sprigs from burning when you cook the scallops.

4. Take two of the sprigs of rosemary and place them side by side and then thread 3 scallops on to the bare ends. Do the same with the rest of the sprigs and now cook the scallops over a medium heat for 2 to 3 minutes on each side.

Once the scallops are cooked remove from barbecue and serve them with some basmati rice and slices of lemon.

Recipe 19 – Seafood Kebabs

It is important to make sure that the pieces of fish are the same size as the pieces of vegetable to ensure that everything is cooked evenly.

Ingredients

12 Large Sea Scallops
12 Large Shrimps Peeled And Deveined But With Tails Intact
340grams Of Snapper Or Other Firm Fleshed Fish Cut Into Pieces
340grams Smoked Sausage Cut Into Pieces Same Size As The Fish
½ Red Bell Pepper Cut Into Pieces
½ Green Bell Pepper Cut Into Pieces
120ml Fresh Orange Juice
60ml Olive Oil
2 Tablespoons Apple Cider Vinegar

1 Teaspoon Minced Chipotle Peppers In Adobo Sauce
½ Teaspoon Ground Cumin
¼ Teaspoon Salt
¼ Teaspoon Freshly Ground Black Pepper

Instructions

1. Place the wooden skewers in a shallow dish full of water and leave to soak for 30 minutes.

2. Next in a bowl combine together the orange juice, olive oil, apple cider vinegar, chipotle peppers, cumin, salt and black pepper and set to one side.

3. On to the soaked skewers now thread the scallops, shrimps, fish, sausage and peppers. Then place into a shallow roasting dish and pour over them the orange juice mixture and leave to marinate in this mixture for 30 minutes in a refrigerator.

4. Now whilst the kebabs are marinating in the sauce you should start heating up the barbecue so that it is ready for cooking the kebabs. Place the grill 4 to 6 inches above the heat source, as you want to cook the kebabs on a medium to high heat.

5. Before placing the kebabs on the grill of the barbecue brush with some oil and then cook them for about 12 minutes (6 minutes on each side). Whilst the kebabs are cooking brush over any remaining sauce regularly.

Once cooked served with some rice or pasta or a fresh green crispy salad.

Recipe 20 – Ocean Packets

Although in this recipe we recommend you use mussels if you can get hold of clams then use these instead. Each packet contains 439 calories and 15.1g of fat.

Ingredients

32 Mussels In Shells Scrubbed And Bearded

32 Shrimps Deveined But Shells Remaining
32 Sea Scallops
8 Corn On The Cob Cut Into Quarters
32 Large Cherry Tomatoes
118grams Unsalted Butter Melted
1 Tablespoon Freshly Grated Lemon Peel

Instructions

1. Turn on your barbecue and place the grill 6 inches above the heat source, as you want to cook these parcels over a medium heat. Plus don't forget to lightly oil the grill before you place the parcels on them.

2. Whilst the barbecue is heating up in a bowl mix together the butter and the lemon peel.

3. Now take 8 sheets of aluminum foil measuring 12 inches by 12 inches and onto each one place 4 mussels, 4 shrimps and 4 sea scallops. Then also place on top of these a piece of the corn on the cob, 4 tomatoes and then drizzle over the butter mixture.

4. Bring opposite ends of the foil together and fold over several times to seal. However don't fold the parcels too tightly as you need to allow room for steam to build up. Do the same for the ends that are open and when ready place on the barbecue.

5. Leave the parcels on the barbecue for between 15 and 20 minutes or until when you open the parcels to take a peek that the mussels have now opened and the shrimps have turned opaque.

6. To serve simply place each parcel on a place then cut across the diagonal and peel the foil back. Garnish each parcel with ½ teaspoon of freshly chopped chives.

Chapter 3 – Healthy Vegetarian Recipes For The Barbecue

Recipe 1 – Grilled Eggplant with Ricotta Salata

A quick and very easy dish to prepare if you have guests to your barbecue who are vegetarians. However you may find this just as enjoyable and extremely good for you containing only 85 calories per serving and 5g of fat.

Ingredients

2 Eggplants Cut Lengthwise Into ½ Inch Thick Slices
2 Tablespoons Extra Virgin Olive Oil
2 Teaspoons Fresh Oregano Leaves
½ Teaspoon Salt
¼ Teaspoon Coarsely Ground Black Pepper
28grams Ricotta Salata or Feta Cheese Crumbled
2 Plum Tomatoes Cut Into ½ Inch Pieces
Lemon Wedges
Oregano Sprigs For Garnish

Instructions

1. Start up barbecue and place grill 4 to 6 inches above heat source, as you will need to cook the eggplant on a medium to high heat.

2. Whilst the barbecue is heating up into a saucepan heat the oil over a medium heat until it is hot but isn't smoking. Then remove from heat and into the oil put the 2 teaspoons of fresh oregano leaves. Now leave to steep until you are ready to serve the eggplant and Ricotta Salata.

3. Lightly oil each side of the slices of eggplant and then sprinkle over some salt and pepper. Place the eggplant on to the grill of the barbecue and close the lid. Cook the eggplant for between 7 and 10 minutes or until they are tender and brown. Don't forget to turn the eggplant over once during this cooking time.

4. Once the eggplant is cooked transfer to a plate and drizzle with the oregano oil prepared earlier then top off with crumbled Ricotta Salata or Feta cheese and tomatoes. Garnish with the sprigs of oregano and serve with the lemon wedges.

Recipe 2 – Beets on the Grill

Although this may be a very simple dish to prepare it is also very flavorsome and will make a wonderful addition to any barbecue meal. Each serving contains 208 calories and 11.9g of fat.

Ingredients

6 Beets Scrubbed
2 Tablespoons Butter
Salt And Pepper To Taste
6 Sheets Of Aluminum Foil

Instructions

1. Start up the barbecue and set the grill to 4 inches above the heat source, as the beets need to be cooked on a high heat.

2. Take 1 sheet of aluminum foil and brush with oil. Now place a beet on to it with some of the butter and then season with salt and pepper. Then wrap the aluminum foil around the beet. Do the same with the other 5 beets.

3. Once the beets are sealed in the aluminum foil and the barbecue has heated up place the parcels on to the grill and cook them for 30 minutes or until the beets have become tender. Let the beets rest for 5 minutes to cool down a little before then serving.

Recipe 3 – Corn and Pepper Jack Quesadillas

You may be surprised to find that the meat loving guests at your barbecue enjoy these quesadillas as much as your vegetarian ones. Although these may contain 330 calories and 11g of fat they are still a very healthy option to serve.

Ingredients

3 Large Ears Of Corn (Husks And Silks Removed)
4 Low Fat Burrito Size Flour Tortillas
113grams Reduced Fat Monterey Jack Cheese Shredded
120ml Mild Or Medium Hot Salsa
2 Green Onions Thinly Sliced
1 Head Romaine Lettuce Thinly Sliced
1 Tablespoon Olive Oil
1 Tablespoon Cider Vinegar
½ Teaspoon Coarsely Ground Black Pepper
¼ Teaspoon Salt

Instructions

1. Prepare the barbecue for covered direct grilling. Placing the grill 4 to 6 inches above heat source as you will want to cook on a medium to high heat.

2. Take the ears of corn and place on the hot grill rack close the lid and cook them for between 10 and 15 minutes or until they start to turn brown in places. It is important that whilst the corn is cooking you turn it often to prevent it from burning. Then when cooked transfer to a plate and allow to cool so handling them is easier.

3. Once the corn has cooled enough take a sharp knife and cut the kernels away from the core of the corn. Whilst the corn is cooling you can make the salad to go with the quesadillas. In a large bowl place the lettuce with the oil, cider vinegar, salt and pepper and then toss all these ingredients together.

4. Take the tortillas and divide between them evenly the cheese, salsa, green onions and corn on to one half of them. Now fold the other half of the tortilla over the top of the filling and this will make your quesadillas.

5. Place the quesadillas on to the hot barbecue grill which you have lightly oiled first and cook for 1 to 2 minutes or until they have turned brown. Make sure that you turn them over once to ensure that everything is cooked through evenly.

Remove from barbecue onto a chopping board and cut into 3 pieces before then transferring to a clean plate and serving with the lettuce.

Recipe 4 – Vegetarian Burgers

This recipe may use very simple ingredients but still comes out making really tasty burgers that are meat free. It is best however to part cook them before placing on the barbecue as this will then stop them from sticking to the barbecue grill.

Ingredients

3 Tablespoons Extra Virgin Olive Oil
1 Large Onion Finely Chopped
1 Garlic Clove Finely Chopped
300grams Carrots Coarsely Grated
300grams Zucchinis Coarsely Grated
1 ½ Teaspoons Ground Cumin
1 ½ Teaspoons Ground Coriander
4 Tablespoons Reduced Fat Peanut Butter
2 Tablespoons Fresh Coriander Chopped
Pepper To Taste
320grams Fresh Whole Wheat Breadcrumbs
1 Egg Beaten

Instructions

1. In a non stick frying pan heat two tablespoons of oil and add the onion and garlic and cook over a medium heat for 5 minutes or until the onion is soft and starting to turn brown. Stir these ingredients frequently. Once the onions have started to turn soft add the carrot and zucchini and fry for another 10 minutes stirring often until the vegetables have become soft. Then stir in the ground cumin, coriander, peanut butter, fresh coriander and pepper. Remove pan from heat and let it cool slightly.

2. Once the above ingredients have cooled sufficiently into these mix the breadcrumbs and egg. Make sure that everything is combined well as you want all the ingredients to bind together.

When ready divide the mixture into 4 equal portions and make 4 patties.

3. Now start the barbecue up and whilst it is heating up you should fry the vegetable burgers off in a frying pan first just to ensure that they stay together. Once they have started to turn slightly brown remove from pan and let them rest for a while. Then when the barbecue is heated up place them on it and finish off cooking them.

4. Just as you would with a conventional burger serve these in a bun with slices of tomato and onion, lettuce and some mayonnaise.

Recipe 5 – Homemade Black Bean Veggie Burgers

Another very tasty vegetarian burger to try that is also very healthy. These particular burgers only contain 198 calories and 3g of fat.

Ingredients

450ml Can Black Beans Drained And Rinsed
½ Green Bell Pepper Cut Into 2 Inch Pieces
½ Onion Cut Into Wedges
3 Garlic Cloves Peeled
1 Egg
1 Tablespoon Chilli Powder
1 Tablespoon Cumin
1 Teaspoon Thai Chilli Sauce Or Hot Sauce
120grams Whole Wheat Breadcrumbs

Instructions

1. Start the barbecue up and cover the grill that needs to be 4 inches above the heat source with some aluminum foil that will have to be lightly oiled before cooking begins.

2. Whilst the barbecue is heating up in to a bowl place the black beans and mash with a fork until they become thick and pasty.

3. In a food processor place the pepper, onion and garlic and turn on until they become finely chopped. Remove these ingredients from the processor and stir into the bowl where the mashed beans are.

4. In another small bowl place the egg and chilli powder, cumin and chilli sauce and mix together well. Then stir this mixture into the bean mixture and then start to add the breadcrumbs. Add enough breadcrumbs to the mixture so that although it is sticky it holds together.

5. Now divide the mixture into 4 equal portions and form burger patties. Place these patties on the lightly oiled aluminum foil on the barbecue and cook on each side for about 8 minutes. Serve these in a whole wheat bun with some slices of tomato, onion, lettuce and some type of relish.

Recipe 6 – Grilled Potato Salad with Gherkins and Mustard

The flavor of these small potatoes is enhanced by the honey and mustard. Whilst the crumbled goats cheese on top helps to add a little softness to what is a very delicious vegetarian dish.

Ingredients

Grilled Potato Salad
900grams Small New Potatoes
2 Teaspoon Sea Salt
1 Large Sweet Onion Cut Into 12 Wedges
4 Garlic Cloves Minced
60ml Olive Oil
60ml Apple Cider Vinegar
1 Tablespoon Fresh Parsley Chopped
Pinch Of Cayenne Pepper
Coarsely Ground Black Pepper And Sea Salt To Taste
240grams Mini Gherkins
60grams Small Black Olives
60grams Sundried Tomatoes Chopped
120grams Goats Cheese Crumbled

Green Mustard Dressing

60ml Olive Oil
60ml Apple Cider Vinegar
80ml Mustard With Herbs
1 Tablespoon Honey
Coarsely Ground Black Pepper And Sea Salt To Taste

Instructions

1. Wash the potatoes to ensure that all dirt is removed and place in a large pot then cover with cold water. Bring the water to a rolling boil and add some sea salt. Then reduce the heat to medium to low and simmer the potatoes for 15 to 20 minutes or until they are just becoming tender. Drain the potatoes and then set to one side to cool for 5 to 10 minutes.

2. Once the potatoes have cooled place them in a large bowl and add these the onion, garlic, olive oil, cider vinegar and parsley. Then season them with the cayenne pepper, sea salt and black pepper. Make sure that you mix these ingredients together well to ensure that everything is coated evenly.

3. Whilst the potatoes are cooling this is when you should start the barbecue up. Place the grill about 4 inches above heat source, as you want to cook the potatoes on the barbecue on a high heat.

4. Once the barbecue is ready if you have a grill basket place the potatoes and onions in it. Using this will making turning the potatoes over a lot easier. Grill them for between 10 and 15 minutes making sure that you turn them over regularly to prevent them from burning. Once they are tender and lightly charred remove from the heat.

5. Now transfer the potatoes and onions to a bowl and into this add the gherkins, olives, sundried tomatoes, green onion and parsley and mix well together. Then set to one side whilst you make the mustard dressing.

6. To make the mustard dressing place in a small bowl the olive oil, cider vinegar, mustard and honey and whisk. Season with some coarsely ground black pepper and sea salt to taste.

7. Take the bowl of potatoes and place on a serving plate then pour over the mustard dressing. Toss the potatoes and other salad ingredients gently to ensure that everything is now coated in the dressing then just before serving crumble over the goat's cheese.

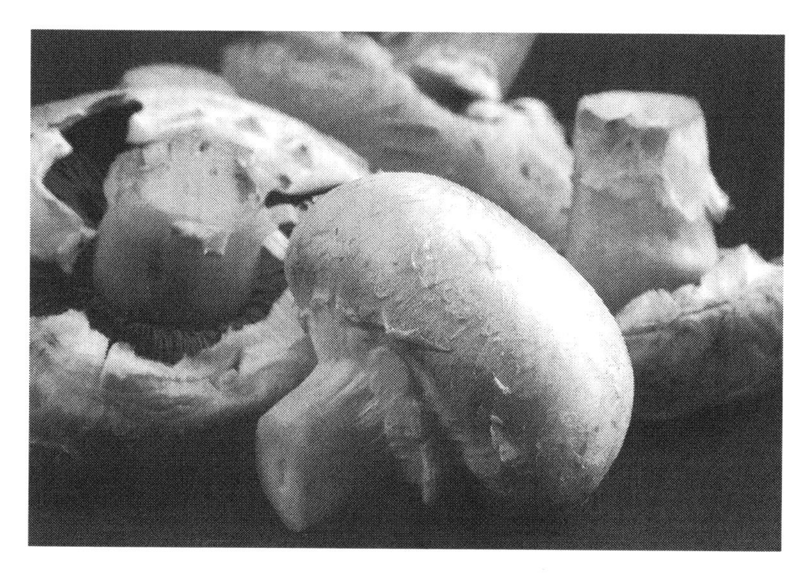

Recipe 7 – Portobello Mushrooms, Goat Cheese and Walnut Sliders

If you are looking for something small to serve at your barbecue that is also meat free then look no further than this recipe. Each one of these sliders contains 198 calories and 11g of fat.

Ingredients

4 Portobello Mushroom Caps
1 Small Onion Thinly Sliced And Caramelized
2 Teaspoon Vegetable Oil
2 Tablespoon Fresh Chives Finely Chopped
80grams Walnuts Finely Chopped
½ Teaspoon Salt
½ Teaspoon Freshly Ground Black Pepper

125grams Goat Cheese (Room Temperature)
Olive Oil

Instructions

1. Start off by caramelizing the onions to do this place them in a saucepan with some vegetable oil and cook for about 15 to 20 minutes. Once the onions are caramelized remove from heat and set to one side for use later.

2. In a small bowl mix together the chives, walnuts, salt and pepper and place this mixture then on to the surface of a chopping board.

3. Take the goats cheese out of its packaging and roll it over the mixture just made making sure that it coats all the cheese evenly. Then cut the cheese into 8 equal slices. Make sure you clean the knife after each slice has been cut and set these to one side.

4. Remove the stems from the mushrooms and brush off any dirt that may still be there. Then with a spoon very gently remove the gills and then brush both sides of the mushroom with some olive oil then grill them on the barbecue over a medium heat for 4 minutes on the gill side first, before then turning them over and cooking them for a further 3 minutes. Once cooked cut each mushroom in half.

5. Now take each mushroom and place them on the bottom part of a whole wheat roll and on top of this then place a slice of the goat's cheese. Then top this off with the caramelized onions and some lettuce. Then top off with the other part of the bun and serve.

Recipe 8 – Grilled Eggplant Teriyaki

This particular vegetable was just made to be grilled and the Asian style marinade helps to bring out more of the eggplants subtle flavors.

Ingredients

2 Medium Large Eggplants
2 Green Onions (Green Part Only) Thinly Sliced

½ Red Bell Pepper Finely Diced
1 Tablespoon Sesame Seeds

Teriyaki Marinade

60ml Reduced Sodium Soy Sauce
60ml Sake Or White Wine
2 Tablespoons Safflower Oil
2 Teaspoons Dark Sesame Oil
3 Tablespoons Natural Granulated Sugar
2 Tablespoons Rice Vinegar or White Wine Vinegar
1 to 2 Garlic Cloves Minced (Optional)
1 Teaspoon Fresh Ginger Grated

Instructions

1. To make the Teriyaki marinade combine together the soy sauce, sake, safflower oil, sesame oil, sugar, rice vinegar, ginger and garlic. Allow to stand until all the sugar has dissolved. When using this marinade to baste the eggplant make sure that you stir it well to ensure that all ingredients remain combined together.

2. Slice the eggplants into ½ inch thick pieces with the peel intact. Then salt them and let them stand in a colander for 30 minutes as this will help to make them a little softer. After the 30 minutes have elapsed make sure that you rinse the eggplant out well.

3. Heat up your barbecue placing the grill 6 inches above the heat source, as you want to cook the eggplant on a medium heat.

4. Once the barbecue is heated up brush each side of the eggplant with a generous amount of the Teriyaki marinade and place on the barbecue. Grill each side for about 5 to 10 minutes or until each side are nice and brown and the eggplant is tender. Make sure that whilst the eggplant is cooking that you baste it regularly with more of the marinade.

5. As soon as the eggplant is cooked remove from the barbecue and place on a chopping board to cool slightly. Once a little cooler cut the eggplant into strips and place in a serving dish then to the strips add the green onions and stir. Pour over some of the

remaining marinade to help moisten the eggplant and increase the flavor then sprinkle over the top the diced red pepper and sesame seeds. Then serve.

Recipe 9 – Tofu and Potato Kebabs

This is an extremely easy meal to prepare for both vegetarian and vegan guests you invite to your next barbecue.

Ingredients

Kebabs
4 Medium Sized Red Skinned Potatoes
900grams Extra Firm Tofu
2 Medium Sweet Red Bell Peppers Cut Into 1 Inch Pieces
Sweet And Savory Sauce
360ml Tomato Sauce
3 Tablespoons Agave Nectar Or Maple Syrup
1 Tablespoon Molasses
1 Tablespoon Olive Oil
2 Tablespoons Soy Sauce Or Tamari To Taste
1 Teaspoon Sweet Or Smoked Paprika
1 Teaspoon Chilli Powder
1 Teaspoon Dried Oregano Or Basil

Teriyaki Marinade

60ml Reduced Sodium Soy Sauce
60ml Sake Or White Wine
2 Tablespoons Safflower Oil
2 Teaspoons Dark Sesame Oil
3 Tablespoons Natural Granulated Sugar
2 Tablespoons Rice Vinegar or White Wine Vinegar
1 to 2 Garlic Cloves Minced (Optional)
1 Teaspoon Fresh Ginger Grated

Instructions

1. Cook the potatoes in the microwave or oven until they are done, but are still quite firm. Allow them to cool before then cutting into 1 inch chunks.

2. Take the tofu and cut into ¾ to 1 inch thick slices and press then cut into ¾ to 1 inch dices. Marinate them either in a Teriyaki or Sweet and Savory Sauce for 30 minutes. To make either sauce place all the ingredients listed in a bowl and mix well together then add to them the diced tofu. You could of course place half the diced tofu in the Teriyaki marinade and the other half in the sweet and savory sauce.

3. Whilst the tofu is marinating you should get the barbecue going. Place the grill 6 inches above the heat source so that you can cook the kebabs on a medium heat.

4. Once the tofu is ready remove from marinade and then alternately thread it on to a skewer with chunks of potato and red pepper. After thread the skewers now lightly oil the grill and place the kebabs on it. After placing the kebabs on the grill brush them with some of the remaining sauce and cook them for about 10 minutes in total.

Make sure that you turn them frequently to prevent them burning and also make sure that you regularly brush them with any remaining sauce. Once cooked serve to your guests with a salad or some rice.

Recipe 10 – Grilled Portobello Mushrooms Popeye Club Sandwich

Portobello mushrooms are a staple diet of many vegetarians' diets and have quite a meaty texture to them.

Ingredients

4 Large Portobello Mushroom Caps (Gills Remove And Then Lightly Rinsed And Patted Dry To Remove Any Residue Dirt)
2 Medium Sized Zucchini Trimmed And Cut Lengthwise Into ¼ Inch Thick Slices
2 Large Red Bell Peppers Cut Into Quarters
1 Medium Sized Onion Cut Into ¼ Inch Thick Slices
120ml Port Wine Or Dry Red Wine or Vegetable Broth
3 Tablespoons Soy Sauce
1 ½ Teaspoons Dried Rosemary

1 ½ Teaspoons Dried Parsley
1 ½ Teaspoons Dried Thyme
3 Garlic Cloves Minced
2 Tablespoons Tomato Ketchup
80ml Olive Oil Divided
Salt And Freshly Ground Black Pepper To Taste

To Serve

4 Individual Ciabatta Rolls
240ml Vegan Pesto
700grams Fresh Baby Spinach

Instructions

1. In a shallow dish mix together the wine/broth, soy sauce, dried herbs, garlic, ketchup and 1 tablespoon of olive oil. Then season with some salt and pepper.

2. To this mixture now add the mushrooms and slices of zucchini. Turn them over to make sure that they are well covered in the sauce and leave them to marinate in it for 15 minutes.

3. Whilst the mushrooms and zucchini are marinating get the barbecue going and place the grill 6 inches above the heat source.

4. Take the ciabatta rolls and cut in half and scoop some of the bread inside out to allow you to then create room for the filling. Now brush the cut sides of each ½ of the rolls with 2 or 3 tablespoons of olive and then place on the grill cut side down. Leave them on the grill for about 2 or 3 minutes or until the cut side has started to turn golden brown. Then remove from barbecue and set to one side for use later.

5. Now place the mushrooms, zucchini, peppers and onions on the barbecue grill, which has been lightly oiled, and cook for about 5 minutes on each side. Don't allow the vegetables to dry out as they cook. In fact remove the vegetables as soon as they are cooked.

6. To make the sandwiches you take one half of the roll and spread on this some of the vegan pesto before then layering the

vegetables on top evenly then apply a layer of fresh spinach before then putting the top of the roll on this. Then serve to your guests.

Recipe 11 – Cilantro and Lime Grilled Tofu

The cilantro and lime helps to make the tofu taste even more delicious.

Ingredients

400grams Firm Tofu
60ml Fresh Lime Juice
1 Tablespoon Olive Oil
5 Tablespoons Fresh Cilantro Chopped
2 Garlic Cloves Minced
2 Teaspoons Chilli Powder
¼ Teaspoon Cayenne Pepper
Salt And Freshly Ground Black Pepper To Taste

Instructions

1. Remove tofu from packaging and place on a plate. Now place another plate on top and weigh it down with something weight at least 3 pounds. A large bowl filled with water will work well. Leave the tofu like this for 20 to 30 minutes and then drain off and discard any liquid that has accumulated on the bottom plate.

2. Remove the tofu from the plate and slice lengthwise into 4 thick slabs before then cutting into tubes and threading on to skewers. Now place these skewers on a plate and set aside ready for cooking later.

3. In a bowl whisk together the lime juice, olive oil, cilantro, garlic, chilli powder and cayenne pepper. Then add a little salt and pepper to taste. Then brush this mixture over the tofu and cover them with plastic wrap before leaving them to marinate for at least 2 hours in the refrigerator. If possible leave the tofu kebabs to marinate in the sauce overnight, as they will absorb more of the flavors of it.

4. Once the barbecue is hot enough and after lightly oiling the grill, which is set 6 inches above the heat source, place the tofu kebabs

on the grill. Cook them on a medium heat for between 10 to 15 minutes or until they start to go black in certain places. Make sure that you turn the kebabs over frequently and also brush them regularly in any of the remaining marinade.

5. As soon as the kebabs are cooked place on a clean plate and serve to your guests.

Recipe 12 – Parmesan Roasted Corn on the Cob

It isn't only the vegetarian guests who are invited to your barbecue who will enjoy this particular recipe, so will your other guests. Be aware however that each serving contains 373 calories along with 25.2g of fat due to the use of the Parmesan cheese.

Ingredients

5 Ears Of Corn Husks And Silks Removed
120ml Mayonnaise
240grams Parmesan Cheese Shredded
1 Tablespoon Chilli Powder
1 Teaspoon Salt
1 Teaspoon Freshly Ground Black Pepper

Instructions

1. Get the barbecue heated up and place the grill at a heat that allows you to cook the corn on a medium to high heat. Make sure that before you place the corn on the grill you lightly oil it first to prevent them from sticking to it.

2. Take the mayonnaise and brush it lightly over each ear of corn and then sprinkle over them the shredded Parmesan cheese, chilli powder, salt and pepper. Then wrap each ear in some aluminum foil and then place these on the grill.

3. Leave them on the grill to cook for about 10 minutes making sure that you turn them regularly to prevent them from burning, but not from preventing the kernels turning brown. As soon as the kernels have lost a lot of their firmness and turned light brown remove from barbecue and serve.

Recipe 13 – Grilled Halloumi Kebabs

Halloumi is a wonderful cheese that when cooked correctly retains much of its shape. However it can be quite a salty cheese.

Ingredients

Kebabs
250grams Halloumi Cut Into 24 Cubes
150grams Focaccia Cut Into 12 Cubes
2 Courgettes Sliced With A Speed Peeler Into 12 Ribbons
1 Red Pepper Trimmed Deseeded And Cut Into 12 Pieces
12 Cherry Tomatoes
Olive Oil

Marinade

2 Garlic Cloves Finely Chopped
4 Spring Onions Thinly Sliced On The Diagonal
1 Small Red Chilli Finely Chopped
10 Sprigs Of Coriander Including Stalks Finely Chopped
10 Mint Leaves Finely Chopped
60ml Extra Virgin Olive Oil
3 Lemons

Instructions

1. Make the marinade by mixing together in a bowl the garlic, spring onions, chilli, coriander, mint, olive oil and juice from the 3 lemons.

2. To this mixture now add the cubes of Halloumi and focaccia and cover the bowl with cling before placing in the refrigerator for 1 hour. 20 minutes before you remove the Halloumi from the refrigerator get the barbecue going.

3. After removing the Halloumi from the refrigerator get some skewers and start to thread the chunks of Halloumi and focaccia on to them. Start off threading on a piece of the focaccia and then a cube of Halloumi followed by a ribbon of courgette so it resembles

a spring. Follow this with another piece of the Halloumi and finish each kebab off with a piece of pepper and a tomato.

4. Once the kebabs are ready place on the barbecue grill which is 6 inches above the heat source and which has been lightly oiled and cook for 5 to 10 minutes or until they have started to turn a golden brown. Remember to turn the kebabs often to prevent them burning. Serve immediately with some warm bread and a crisp green salad.

Recipe 14 – Stuffed Peppers on Barbecue

Take your stuffed to a whole new level with this recipe. The barbecue helps to really give the peppers a smoky flavor that complements the cheeses well. Each pepper contains 378 calories and 21g of fat.

Ingredients

3 Red And 3 Yellow Peppers
2 Tablespoons Olive Oil
50gram Pine Nuts
140gram Long Grain Rice
2 Garlic Cloves Chopped
350gram Vegetable Stock
1 Bunch Spring Onions Thinly Sliced
140grams Cherry Tomatoes Halved
150grams Mozzarella Chopped
140grams Gorgonzola
Handful Of Fresh Parsley And Basil Chopped

String For Tying

Instructions

1. To make the filling for the peppers heat the oil in a pan with a lid and fry the pine nuts until they are lightly toasted. To this then add the rice and fry until the grains turn glossy. Then stir in the garlic, add the stock and bring all these ingredients to the boil.

2. Cover the pan and allow the ingredients to cook for 10 minutes until rice becomes tender. Then remove from heat and allow to cool slightly before stirring in the spring onions, tomatoes, mozzarella, Gorgonzola and the fresh parsley and basil. Season with salt and pepper then leave to cool further.

3. To stuff the peppers first cut around the stalk and remove and set aside. Now make one slit down one side and open it out gently. Remove all seeds and membrane. Now spoon in some of the filling left cooling. Take care not to put in too much.

4. Take around a metre of kitchen string and wrap around the centre part of the pepper a couple of times then around the stalk of the pepper which you have replaced and tie of the string firmly. Do this for all six peppers.

5. To cook the peppers place on the grill of the barbecue that has been set 6 inches above the heat source for 15 to 20 minutes. Whilst the peppers are cooking over a medium heat turn them regularly to prevent them from burning. Don't be too concerned if the peppers start to split, just wrap them in some aluminum foil to finish off cooking. Once cooked serve to your guests.

Recipe 15 – Hot Dressed Sweet Potato, Fennel and Feta Parcels

Don't be too surprised if your guests ask you for this recipe. All ingredients used in this recipe complement each other wonderfully.

Ingredients

1 Sweet Potato Peeled And Cut Into Wedges
½ Small Fennel Bulb Sliced
1 Tablespoon Fresh Orange Plus Zest
1 Tablespoon Olive Oil
2 Teaspoon Red Wine Vinegar
1 Teaspoon Runny Honey
1 Tablespoon Flat Leaf Parsley Chopped
1 Tablespoon Walnuts Roughly Chopped
50grams Feta Cheese Crumbled

Instructions

1. On to two pieces of aluminum foil measuring 30cm square place the sweet potato wedges and the fennel. Then pour on 1 teaspoon of orange juice and 1 teaspoon of olive oil and move around to ensure that the sweet potato wedges and fennel are well coated.

2. Now bring up the sides of the aluminum foil to create a bowl and then scrunch the top to seal the vegetables inside. Place the parcel on to the grill of the barbecue over a medium heat and cook for between 35 to 45 minutes or until the potatoes are soft. To test the potatoes unwrap and see if the point of a knife inserts into them easily.

3. Whilst the potatoes and fennel are cooking in a bowl whisk together the rest of the orange juice, olive oil, vinegar, honey, parsley, walnuts and orange zest. Add some salt and pepper to season. Set to one side for use later.

4. When the potatoes and fennel are cooked remove from barbecue open up the parcel and pour in the dressing you made earlier along with most of the crumbled feta. Not only will the heat from the food help to bring out the dressings flavors but also warm the feta up. Gently mix all these ingredients together before then scattering the remaining feta over the top. Serve either in the aluminum foil or on a clean plate with some crusty bread.

Chapter 4 – Healthy Dessert Recipes for the Barbecue

Recipe 1 – Grilled Peaches with Gingersnaps

This particular recipe really helps to make a wonderful end to a fantastic barbecue. Each serving of this meal contains 155 calories and 3.4g of fat.

Ingredients

4 x Firm Peaches Halved And Pitted
4 Teaspoon Canola Oil
8 Tablespoons Brown Sugar
16 Scoops Fat Free Vanilla Yogurt
8 Gingersnap Cookies Crumbled

Instructions

1. These peaches need to be cooked on a high heat so set the grill 4 inches above the heat source. Before you place the peach halves on the grill make sure you brush it with oil first.

2. Take each peach halve and then brush each side of them with the canola oil and then place them on the barbecue grill. Cook the peach halves until they are tender and warmed through which should take around 10 minutes. Turn them over several times to prevent the peaches from burning.

3. When the peaches have become soft remove from barbecue and place on a plate skin side down. Sprinkle with the brown sugar allowing time for it to melt. Then in each half place two scoops of the yogurt and sprinkle the crumbled gingersnap cookies over the top.

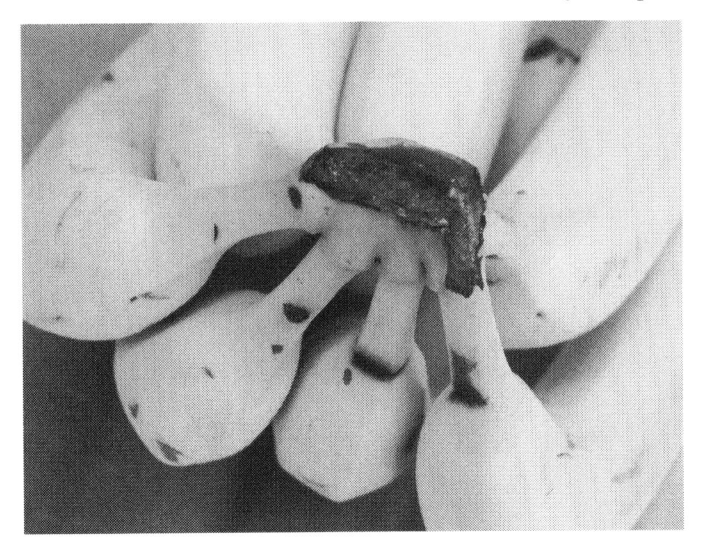

Recipe 2 – Campfire Banana Splits

Anyone who went camping when they were young would have enjoyed this particular dessert. If you would like to reduce the number of calories in this dessert then omit the marshmallows.

Ingredients

6 Large Bananas Unpeeled But Stems Removed
470grams Semi Sweet Chocolate Chips
300grams Miniature Marshmallows

Instructions

1. Whilst the barbecue is heating up take four sheets of aluminum foil big enough to wrap around a banana and lightly oil.

2. Slice the peel of the banana from stem to bottom lengthwise. However make sure that you don't slice all the way through. Now gently open the banana up just enough to place some of the chocolate chips and marshmallows inside.

3. Now place on a sheet of aluminum foil and wrap around the banana. Then place on the barbecue grill or if you want directly in to the coals and leave their to cook for about 5 minutes. This

should provide sufficient time for both the marshmallows and chocolate chips to melt.

4. To serve simply unwrap the bananas open them up wide and provide your guests with a spoon. If you want you could provide some fresh frozen vanilla yogurt with them or some vanilla ice cream.

Recipe 3 – Grilled Pineapple

Not only is this dish really easy to prepare and cook but tastes really wonderful as well. The hot sauce helps to give a little kick to the dish as well as cut through some of its sweetness. This particular recipe contains just 46 calories per serving and 2.9g of fat.

Ingredients

1 Fresh Pineapple Peeled Cored And Cut Into 1 Inch Rings
¼ Teaspoon Honey
3 Tablespoons Melted Butter
1 Dash Hot Pepper Sauce
Salt To Taste

Instructions

1. In a resealable bag place the pineapple rings and to this then add the honey, melted butter, hot pepper sauce and salt. Now seal the bag and shake gently to ensure that each piece of pineapple is coated in the sauce evenly.

Place in the refrigerator for at least 30 minutes for the pineapple to marinate in the sauce. However if you want the pineapple to take on even more of the sauce flavor then it is best to leave it marinating overnight.

2. To cook place the grill of the barbecue 4 inches above the heat source and lightly oil the grill. You will want to cook the pineapple on a high heat.

3. As soon as the barbecue is warm enough place the pineapple rings on the barbecue grill and cook on each side for 2 to 3 minutes or until they have become heated through and there are grill marks on the surface. Remove and serve to your guests.

Recipe 4 – Honey Glazed Grilled Plums

Drizzling honey over the plums as they cook not only helps to soften them but also helps to release their own natural juices. Once cooked serve to your guests with a scoop or two of frozen vanilla yogurt. Each serving of this dish contains just 285 calories and 2g of fat.

Ingredients

4 Firm Plums Halved And Pitted
6 Tablespoons Honey
700grams Frozen Vanilla Yogurt To Serve

Instructions

1. Turn on the barbecue and place the grill 6 inches above the heat source, as you will be cooking the plums on a medium heat.

2. Whilst the barbecue is heating up take the 8 halves of plums and in a bowl place them with 2 tablespoons of honey. Toss them very gently to ensure that they are covered in the honey well but to ensure that the plums don't get bruised.

3. Once the barbecue has heated up lightly brush the grill with some oil before then placing the plums on to it flesh side down first. Leave on the grill for about 3 minutes or until they have turned a light brown.

4. Turn the plums over so that they are now skin side down on the grill and allow to cook for a further 2 or 3 minutes or they have become soft and warmed through. Immediately serve them to your guests with some frozen vanilla yogurt.

Recipe 5 – Grilled Peaches

Although a very simple dish to make you will find that this makes a sophisticated end to the barbecue. Even with the adding of blue cheese to the dish each serving only contains 147 calories and 5.2g of fat.

Ingredients

2 Large Fresh Peaches Peeled, Halved And Pitted
3 Tablespoons White Sugar
180ml Balsamic Vinegar
2 Teaspoons Freshly Ground Black Peppercorns
70grams Blue Cheese Crumbled

Instructions

1. In a saucepan over a medium heat mix together the sugar, vinegar and pepper. Let this mixture simmer until it has reduced by half and becomes slightly thicker. Remove from the heat and set to one side for use later.

2. Place the grill on your barbecue 6 inches above the heat source and lightly grill. Now place on it the peach halves cut side down first and cook for about 5 minutes or until the flesh has become caramelized. Now turn the peaches over and brush with the balsamic mixture and cook for a further 2 or 3 minutes.

3. Once cooked remove from barbecue and place in individual serving dishes before then drizzling them with the remainder of the balsamic mixture and sprinkling with the crumbled blue cheese. Then serve to your guests.

Recipe 6 – Grilled Apricots with Brioche and Vanilla Ice Cream

If you are going to try out this recipe then serve them with a crisp dessert wine.

Ingredients

8 Ripe Apricots Halved And Pitted
2 Tablespoons Unsalted Butter Melted
2 Tablespoons Sugar
4 Slices Brioche 1 Inch Thick
2 Tablespoons Warm Honey
475grams Vanilla Ice Cream

Instructions

1. Heat up the barbecue placing the grill 6 inches above the heat source, as you will be cooking the apricots on a medium heat.

2. Whilst the barbecue is heating up drizzle the apricot halves with the melted butter before sprinkling on the sugar. Set to one side for now for cooking later.

3. Take the four slices of brioche and place them on the grill that has been lightly oiled first and cook for a minute on each side.

4. Next take the apricots and place these on to the lightly oiled barbecue grill and cook for 2 to 3 minutes on each side. Once cooked transfer them on to clean plates which the slices of brioche have already been placed.

5. To serve drizzle some more honey over the apricots and brioche before then topping off each apricot half with a scoop of vanilla ice cream.

Recipe 7 – Grilled Fruit Kebabs

This is a great summer dessert and these can be cooking whilst you are enjoying the other food on offer at your barbecue. Each one of these kebabs contains 268 calories and 15.4g of fat.

Ingredients

120grams Margarine
60ml Honey
3 Fresh Peaches Pitted And Quartered
3 Fresh Plums Pitted And Quartered
3 Bananas Peeled And Cut Into 4 Pieces Each

12 Strawberries Hulled

Instructions

1. On to your preheated barbecue grill place a large sheet of aluminum foil.

2. In a small saucepan melt together the margarine and honey over a medium heat. Once the margarine has melted completely reduce the heat to low and cook gently until the mixture has become slightly thicker. This should take about 5 minutes and whilst it is cooking make sure that you stir the mixture occasionally. Remove from heat and leave to one side for use later.

3. Take the skewers (if they are wooden ones remember to soak them in a bowl of water for at least 30 minutes to prevent them from burning). On to these start to thread the pieces of fruit. Start with a piece of peach followed by a piece of plum and a piece of banana and end of each kebab with a strawberry.

4. Once all fruit kebabs are made place them on the aluminum foil and then spoon over the honey and margarine mixture. Cook the kebabs until the fruit has become softened and the sauce coating them has thickened and cooked onto the fruit. This should take around 5 minutes. Now flip the skewers and spoon over some more of the sauce and cook for another 5 minutes. Once cooked serve to your guests immediately.

Recipe 8 – Simple Grilled Pineapple Milhojas

This is a very popular dessert in Argentina and includes the use of a form of caramel known as "Dulce de Leche". The caramel sauce is easy to make but can also be purchased ready made. Each serving of this particular dessert contains 495 calories and 25g of fat.

Ingredients

12 Pineapple Rings
3 Sheets Puff Pastry
2 x 140ml Cans Sweetened Condensed Milk
570ml Citrus Sorbet Of Your Choice

Instructions

1. The first thing you need to do is make the "Dulce de Leche". To do this take the tins of condensed milk remove all labels and place the unopened tins into a large saucepan. Now pour in enough water to cover the tins by at least 1 or 2 inches and bring the water to boil over a high heat. Then reduce the heat and cover the saucepan and leave the tins to simmer in the water for 3 hours.

After 3 hours drain all water away remove cans from saucepan and leave the tins to then cool to room temperature before you open them.

2. Whilst the tins are in the water take the sheets of puff pastry and cook as per the instructions provided then leave to one side to cool.

3. After removing the "Dulce de Leche" from the tins pour half of it over the first sheet of cooked puff pastry and then top with a second sheet of puff pastry. Then pour the rest of the "Dulce de Leche" over this sheet before topping off with the third one. Now cut into 12 triangles.

4. Over a medium heat on the barbecue take the slices of pineapple and grill them until they have warmed through and become nicely marked. Remember to turn them once during this cooking time.

5. Once the pineapple is cooked take a slice of the puff pastry and "Dulce de Leche" and garnish with a grilled pineapple ring and a scoop of sorbet and serve them to your guests.

Recipe 9 – Red Hot Apples

These can be cooking whilst your guests can be enjoying the other food you have presented to them at your barbecue.

Ingredients

4 Medium Size Tart Apples Cored
4 Teaspoons Brown Sugar

60grams Red Cinnamon Candies

Vanilla Ice Cream To Serve (Optional)

Instructions

1. Take each cored apple and place it on a large piece of heavy duty aluminum foil that has been lightly oiled. Then into the centre of each apple you place a teaspoon of the sugar and 1 tablespoon of the red cinnamon candies. Now fold the foil around the apple and seal tightly.

2. Place these parcels on the grill over a medium to high heat and cook them for 30 minutes or until the apples have become tender.

3. Once cooked very gently transfer the apples and their syrup from the barbecue to plates and open the parcels up. Then if you want place a scoop of ice cream on top of the still warm apples and serve to your guests.

Recipe 10 – Toasty Campfire Cookies

You will find that these are the tastiest cookies you have ever tasted. Don't be surprised if not only the children but also the adults at your next barbecue come back asking for more.

Ingredients

25grams Chopped White Chocolate
20 Oatmeal Cookies
30grams Milk Chocolate Candy
240grams Miniature Marshmallows

Instructions

1. First off melt the white chocolate and then spread this evenly over the bottoms of the cookies.

2. Take the milk chocolate and break up into 10 pieces and then place 1 piece on top of one of the white chocolate covered cookies. Then place the marshmallows on top of this. Take another one of

the cookies with only the white chocolate on and place this on top so making a sandwich.

3. Place the cookies on to the grill of your barbecue and cook until the marshmallows and milk chocolate has begun to melt. This should be about 3 minutes. Remove from heat and serve to your guests.

Recipe 11 – Rum Spiked Grilled Pineapple with Toasted Coconut

The caramelizing of the sugar in this dessert means not only does it taste delicious on its own but also when served with a low fat vanilla ice cream or frozen yogurt. If you wish you can replace the pineapple with firm peaches or apricots.

Ingredients

1 Pineapple Peeled Cored Halved Lengthwise And Then Sliced Into 12 Wedges Lengthwise
60grams Light Brown Sugar
60ml Dark Spiced Rum
1 Tablespoon Butter
2 Tablespoons Sweetened Coconut Toasted

Low Fat Vanilla Ice Cream To Serve (Optional)

Instructions

1. In a microwave safe bowl combine together the sugar and rum. Microwave on high for 1 ½ minutes or until all the sugar has dissolved. Take this mixture and then brush it evenly over all the wedges of pineapple.

2. Take the butter, which you have melted and drizzle this over the pineapple before then placing the wedges on the barbecue grill and cooking over a medium heat for 6 minutes. Turn the wedges over once half way through. Once the pineapple wedges are heated through and have become marked by the grill remove and place on to plates.

3. Now sprinkle over some of the toasted coconut and should you wish add a spoonful of low fat vanilla ice cream to the plate as well.

Recipe 12 – Succulent Grilled Peaches with Honey Chevre

The sweetness of the peaches when warm goes extremely well with the creaminess of the goat's cheese, which is further complemented by a touch of honey. Yet for such a delicious tasting dessert each serving only contains 99 calories and 6.3g of fat.

Ingredients

4 Fresh Peaches Halved And Pitted
170gram Soft Goat Cheese (Chevre)
2 Tablespoons Skimmed Milk
1 Tablespoon Honey
8 Mint Leaves For Garnish

Instructions

1. Preheat the barbecue placing the grill 6 inches above the heat source, as you will be cooking the peaches on a medium heat. Before placing the peaches on the grill make sure you lightly oil it first.

2. In a small bowl combine together the cheese, milk and honey and set to one side. If you want place it in the refrigerator whilst the peaches are cooking.

3. Take the peach halves and place on the grill cut side down so that they begin to caramelize and grill marks begin to appear. Cook them on the cut side for between 5 and 7 minutes.

4. Remove the peaches from the grill and place on to plates to serve to your guests. In each half of peach place a tablespoon of the cheese mixture and then garnish with a mint leaf.

Recipe 13 – Kiwi, Banana and Strawberry Kebabs

It may seem a strange combination, but these kebabs taste absolutely delicious.

Ingredients

2 Kiwi Fruit Peeled And Quartered
3 Bananas Peeled And Cut Into Thick Slices
12 Strawberries Hulled But Left Whole
1 Tablespoon Fresh Lemon Juice
1 Teaspoon Ground Mixed Spice
2 Tablespoons Melted Butter
2 Tablespoons Maple Syrup

Instructions

1. In a bowl place the lemon juice, mixed spice, melted butter and maple syrup and mix well together. Now place to one side ready for when you start cooking the kebabs.

2. On to four skewers thread 3 strawberries, some banana slices and some kiwi fruit. Make sure that you thread each fruit on to the skewers alternately.

3. Once the skewers are ready place on the preheated barbecue with the grill placed 6 inches above the heat source, as you want to cook them on a medium heat. Cook each kebab for 1 to 2 minutes on each side making sure that you regularly brush over the maple syrup mixture. Once they have turned a golden brown serve immediately to your guests.

Recipe 14 – Honey Barbecued Figs

Figs lend themselves well to being cooked on a barbecue and the honey helps to bring out the rich flavor of these fruit even more.

Ingredients

12 Large Ripe Figs
4 Tablespoons Honey

2 Tablespoons White Wine

Instructions

1. Into a small saucepan place the honey and wine and heat making sure that you stir it continuously until the ingredients become well blended. If you want you can actually do this process on the barbecue.

2. Now take the figs and cut these in half lengthways and then brush them with the honey mixture and place on the barbecue grill. Cook them over a low to medium heat for around 5 minutes and keep basting them with any of the honey mixture you have left over. To cook on a low to medium heat place the grill of the barbecue 6 to 8 inches above the heat source.

Recipe 15 – Chocolate Stuffed Bananas

As children we loved these and certainly as adults we can enjoy them as well.

Ingredients

4 Medium Bananas
125grams (24 Squares) Milk Chocolate
Whipped Cream Or Low Fat Frozen Vanilla Yogurt To Serve

Instructions

1. Take each banana and cut lengthways through the skin making sure that you don't cut all the way through the bottom layer of the bananas skin.

2. Now into the cut made you should place 6 squares of the milk chocolate.

3. Take a piece of aluminum foil and wrap this around each of the bananas and place them on the barbecue grill 6 inches above the heat source. Cook over a medium heat for 10 minutes, making sure that you turn them over half way through.

4. Once the cooking time is up remove the parcels from the barbecue and then remove the bananas from the foil before placing on to plates and serving with a bowl of whipped cream or low fat frozen vanilla yogurt.

MORE 70 BEST EVER RECIPES EBOOKS REVEALED AT MY AUTHOR PAGE:-

CLICK HERE TO ACCESS THEM NOW

Printed in Great Britain
by Amazon

61385511R00056